# HOME SCHOOL FAMILY FITNESS

The Complete Physical Education
Curriculum Guide for Grades K–12

## DR. BRUCE WHITNEY

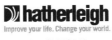
Improve your life. Change your world.

NEW YORK

Exercise illustrations © Sarah Stern
Diagrams by Anna Krusinski

Hatherleigh Press is committed to preserving and protecting the natural resources of the Earth. Environmentally responsible and sustainable practices are embraced within the company's mission statement.

Hatherleigh Press is a member of the Publishers Earth Alliance, committed to preserving and protecting the natural resources of the planet while developing a sustainable business model for the book publishing industry.

PEA Member     Recycled Content

Recycled Content: This book is printed on 20% recycled paper, of which 10% is derived from postconsumer waste.

**hatherleigh**

5–22 46th Avenue, Suite 200
Long Island City, NY 11101
www.hatherleighpress.com

CIP data available upon request

ISBN 978-1-57826-274-8
*Home School Family Fitness* is available for bulk purchase, special promotions, and premiums. For information on reselling and special purchase opportunities, call 1–800–528–2550 and ask for the Special Sales Manager.

*Interior design by Beth Kessler, Neuwirth & Associates, Inc.*
*Cover design by Pauline Neuwirth, Neuwirth & Associates, Inc.*

42

Printed in the United States

# ACKNOWLEDGEMENTS

MY HEARTFELT THANKS goes to physical therapist Sherrie Lange, whose counsel on the exercises was invaluable.

This book would not be possible without my wife, Lynn, and our nine children, who tested games, created drills and games, and endured being "guinea pigs." Their input from a child's perspective was essential.

*I would like to dedicate this
book to my wonderful Creator, who
has created our bodies with amazing
detail and has given us the responsibility
to properly take care of them.*

# TABLE OF CONTENTS

# QUICK START WITH WEEKLY LESSON PLANS

TO MAXIMIZE THE potential of this book and to develop a personalized physical education curriculum program for your child, you will need to read all the chapters of this book. If you do not want to take the time to read this book, however, you can begin with a "Quick Start."

## QUICK START

Below is a series of tasks that you can add to your "to do" list right away to help you get started. This shortcut is intended to help you get started, and as you gain confidence, you can begin to customize the items in this book for your family and lifestyle. I recommend adding one of these points each week, so you will not feel overwhelmed. Once you cover all these points with your student, you will have a well-rounded physical education program covering the major areas: muscle strength, aerobics, and sports skills. Plus, you will have fun together!

- Photocopy "Height and Weight" page in the Appendix. Record the children's height and weight on a monthly basis.
- Read Chapter 2: Muscle Strength and Endurance. Photocopy the "Muscle Strength and Endurance" chart and put it on your fridge. Get your children started on a muscle-strengthening program, and have the children record the exercises they do on the chart for accountability.
- Use the **Weekly Lesson Plans** below.

- Each week, set aside one recess period to teach your children two new games from chapter 4.
- Use any of the games from chapter 4 for birthday parties.
- Assign the children to teach neighborhood children any of the games from chapter 4.
- Read chapter 3: Aerobics. Photocopy the labs on pages 35 to 37. Have the children do the labs and begin the exercise journal page 40.
- Skim chapter 6: Lesson Plans. The lesson plans are designed to become progressively more challenging. I encourage you to start all children with the first plan and progress from there. Feel free to move quickly through the units that are easy for your child, and spend more time on those that are difficult.
- Skim Chapter 7: Labs. With the help of these pages, you as a parent can teach advanced sport skills with confidence—even if you cannot perform the skill yourself. In fact, if you perform a skill poorly, your child can critique you and actually learn *more* about how the skill is performed. Note that as a home school family, if you complete the labs together, your child will have received better instruction than in a typical gym class because of the personal instruction received.

**Will your child** do better in math if he is physically fit?

See page xxi for the answer.

**Children in grades** 4 and above are capable of teaching each other from the lab sheets. First and second graders will not have the coordination or strength to successfully do all the labs, but they can still have fun trying.

## WEEKLY LESSON PLANS

Below is a suggested list of activities. A typical school year has 36 weeks of instruction, and I have 40 weeks of instruction listed. If you need to skip a week, such as week 18 because you have no snow, you should still have more than enough activities to take you through the school year.

I recommend you do physical education activities between 3 to 5 days per week.

**Physical education instruction** is required by law in 45 states. Details vary from state to state. Public schools typically give instruction in physical education twice a week for 30 minutes a day. In addition to this, students typically have a minimum of 30 minutes per day of unstructured recess play time.

I recommend you schedule one hour of instruction per week for your home.

## Week 1 (September)

**K–12**

♦ Do **Fitness Test** (chapter 5): Mark off a 1-mile course. Put a chalk mark on the road by the front wheel where you begin, drive your car around the block, stop when your odometer is at one mile, and put a chalk mark by the front wheel.

♦ Memorize the major bones of the body on page 11.

## Week 2

**K–12**

• Do these exercises from 10 a.m.–10:15 a.m., during a "morning exercise break:" Roll-Up, Push-up, Pull-up, Kangaroo Jumps, and Flying exercises (see chapter 2).

• Duplicate page 23, Muscle Strength and Endurance Log one per student.

• Football page 117 and do Football Punt and Catch page 121.

• Take the written test on bones of the body page 25.

## Week 3

**Pre-school–Grade 3** Do Walking, Running, and Jumping Lesson page 76.

**Grades 4–12**

• Start the aerobics program in chapter 3. Duplicate pages 35–37 one per student.

• Soccer page 107 and game #6 Speedy Soccer page 51.

• Memorize the major muscles of the body on page 12.

## Week 4

**Pre-school–Grade 12** Jump Rope Lesson page 92. Do Tiger Tails page 47 and Four Square page 44. Take the written test on muscles of the body page 24.

## Week 5

**Pre-school–Grade 3** Many Ways of Moving Lesson page 77.

**Grades 4–12** Do Speedy Soccer page 51.

## Week 6

**Pre-school–Grade12** Indoor Mini-basketball page 46 and Lightning Basketball page 52.

**Grades 4–12** Basketball page 125.

## Week 7

**Pre-school–Grade 3** Beanbag and Movement Lesson page 78.

**Grades 4–12** Do Kids' Handball page 52.

## Week 8

**Pre-school–Grade 3** Hoops and Movement Lesson page 79.

**Grades 4–12** Do Lightning Basketball page 46.

## Week 9

**Pre-school–Grade 12** Ball-Handling Lesson (Throw, Catch, Dribble, Bounce) page 80.

## Week 10

**Pre-school–Grade 12** Ball Handling Lesson (Striking and Kicking a ball) page 82.

## Week 11

**Pre-school–Grade 12** Paddle Ball Lesson page 83

HOME SCHOOL FAMILY FITNESS

## Week 12

**Pre-school–Grade 12** Soccer Lead-up Activities Lesson page 83

## Week 13

**Pre-school–Grade 12** Basketball Lead-up Activities Lesson page 83

## Week 14

**Pre-school–Grade 12** Dance Lesson p. 96 Library music required. Juggling page 84

## Week 15

**Pre-school–Grade 12** Basic Elementary Stunts Lesson page 85

## Week 16

**Pre-school–Grade 12** Basic Elementary Stunts Lesson page 85

## Week 17

**Pre-school–Grade 12** Swimming Unit page 88 (I encourage a family outing but you may choose to skip this unit.)

## Week 18

**Pre-school–Grade 12** Snow Games page 56 (If you have no snow, you may skip this unit.)

## Week 19

**Pre-school–Grade 2** Do Simon Says page 44 and Follow The Leader page 44
**Grades 1–12** Do Dodgeball page 46

## Week 20

**Pre-school–Grade 12**

* Add Baseball exercises Pre-Throwing 1 and Pre-Throwing 2 page 18–19 to your daily 10 a.m. exercise time.
* Do Tug of War page 53 Standoff page 12

## Week 21

**Pre-school–Grade 12** Do Freeze Tag page 53 and Lab: Walking and Running Correctly page 103

## Week 22

**Pre-school–Grade 2** Do Balloon Volleyball page 45
**Grades 3–12** Do Deck Tennis page 52 and Floor Tennis page 47

## Week 23

**Pre-school–Grade 12** Do Pin Guard page 46 and Aerobic Ball Exercises page 163

## Week 24

**Pre-school–Grade 4** Do Badminiature page 47
**Grades 4–12** Do Snake Catch p. 54 and Anti-I-Over page 49

## Week 25

**Pre-school–Grade 2** Ball Handling Lesson page 80
**Grades 2–12** Do 500 Baseball page 50

## Week 26

**Pre-school–Grade 2** Ball Handling Lesson page 80

**Grades 3–12** Four Square page 44

## Week 27

**Pre-school–Grade 4** Hopscotch page 45

**Grades 3–12** Home Run Baseball page 50. Do Baseball Labs pages 142–144

## Week 28

**Pre-school–Grade 12** Kickball page 50

## Week 29

**Pre-school–Grade 12** Speedy Soccer page 51

**Grades 4–12** do Soccer Labs page 114–117

## Week 30

**Pre-school–Grade 12** Newcomb Volleyball page 51

**Grades 4–12** do Volleyball Labs page 148–150

## Week 31

**Pre-school–Grade 12** Freeze Tag page 53

## Week 32

**Pre-school–Grade 12** Dodgeball page 46

## Week 33

**Pre-school–Grade 12** game Forty Ways to Get There page 44

**Grades 4–12** Tennis Labs page 153–156

## Week 34

**Pre-school–Grade 3** Blanket Toss page 46

**Grades 3–12** Frisbee Football page 51

## Week 35

Post Fitness Tests Chapter 5

## Week 36

**Pre-school–Grade 12** Cops and Robbers page 53

## Week 37

**Pre-school–Grade 12** Kid's Handball page 52

## Week 38

**Pre-school–Grade 12** Do a family bike trip of 3 miles.

## Week 39

**Pre-school–Grade 12** Do a family hike of 2 miles.

## Week 40

Invite another family over to play kickball.

**AUTHOR'S NOTE:**

Further visual reference for this book, including photographs of my children participating in many of the exercises and activities, can be found on my website, www.HSFFI.com. The website also provides information on how to order my DVD, which demonstrates the drills and games in Chapter 7: Rules and Teaching Labs for Sports.

# INTRODUCTION

NOT LONG AGO I was at a graduation party with Becky and her husband, good friends of mine whom I have known for several years. Both Becky and her husband are church youth workers. As we chatted, Becky asked if she could get my opinion on something. She wanted my assessment on a youth-related topic since I have taught and coached children for over 20 years.

She said, "Bruce, I am alarmed by the increase in the number of overweight children I supervise during the past three decades. It's showing up at a younger and younger age—even lower elementary children are overweight! Have you noticed the same trend?"

Her question got me thinking. I began to informally quiz other friends of mine: everyone from nurses, to educators and religious workers. Since I am a physical education major, many of my friends often consult me when they are concerned for the health and fitness of children they know. This time, when I asked them about kids and obesity they all agreed: the children they knew were gaining more weight and were less fit.

If this is true, I thought, then this is a serious problem that needs to be addressed.

But first, I wanted to know more about the facts, so I began to do some research. The information I uncovered confirmed my suspicions—except it was even worse than I thought.

Since then, I have felt personally and professionally compelled to do everything possible to change this trend towards unfit and unhealthy youth.

But I need help from you, the parent. Let's look at the facts together.

## THE BOTTOM LINE:

Over the past 40 years, individuals in our society have become more sedentary, less fit, and increasingly overweight. The recipe of an inactive lifestyle, low fitness level, and overweight body type add up to a dangerous reality.

### What is fitness?

Fitness refers to the health of the body and the ability to perform a variety of physical activities. The profession of physical education typically measures a child's fitness health by testing five different components of the body. These components include:

- Cardio-respiratory endurance (heart and lungs)
- Body composition (percentage of body fat)
- Muscular strength
- Muscular endurance
- Flexibility of muscles

An individual who is not physically fit is unhealthy in one or all of the above categories, and is endangering the health of his or her entire body.

## Overweight Trends Among Children in the U.S.

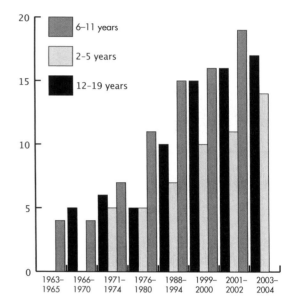

Our children are less active today than ever before.

**Children ages 8 to 18** spend an average of 6.5 hours a day doing what we call *"consuming media"* (that is, watching TV, playing video games, watching DVDs, listening to or downloading music, and surfing the internet or playing games on the computer).[1]

The bottom line is, our children are spending more time in front of a TV screen or a computer screen, and less time engaging in active recreational activities.

1  Kaiser Family Foundation, "Generation M: Media in the Lives of 8–18 Year-Olds," 2005.

**California as a Case Study**

In 1995, California began mandatory fitness testing for public school children, using the Fitnessgram test. (This exam has become the new national standard fitness test and is now mandatory for students in Texas, Alabama, Delaware, California, South Carolina, West Virginia, and many individual school districts like New York City and Miami-Dade County schools). **California is the only state to publish the test results; therefore, we must look to them as an example.** In 2007, 70.6% of California's students failed to meet state standards for all-around healthy physical fitness. California has seen small improvements in the fitness level of the school age children but has a long way to go.

| 2003 | 2004 | 2005 | 2006 | 2007 |
|------|------|------|------|------|
| 75.3 | 73 | 73.3 | 72.5 | 70.6 |

Percentage of California students who fail to meet the states all-around-physical fitness standards (461,404 students tested)

If we believe California's half-million students tested to be representative of all U.S. children, it is clear that the decline in physically fit children is alarming.

## Ask yourself . . .

Are you unintentionally promoting sedentary activity by not offering your child an alternative to playing video games or watching TV?

As parents, we need to limit our children's sedentary activities, like time in front of a TV or computer screen, and make sure that adequate physical activity is part of their lives.

**The average 6- to 11-year-old** watches 20 hours of television a week.

## FITNESS

Not only do we need to encourage our children to be active, we also need to help them become fit—for life. This means following an exercise regimen.

Ask parents and teachers if children are physically fit and the general answer is, "No—and they are less fit than ever before!" What do the facts have to say?

According to a fitness survey by the President's Council on Physical Fitness and Sport from 1999, half of all U.S. school children do not participate in enough exercise to maintain their heart and lung systems.

## OVERWEIGHT

Poor performance in school fitness programs and an inactive lifestyle increase the odds of becoming overweight.

The term *overweight* means that an individual has a higher percentage of body fat than what is recommended for their age range and gender. In the United States, the number of overweight children ages 6 to 11 has increased 400% from 1963 to 2000. From ages 12 to 19, the number of overweight children has increased 300%. [2]

The graph on page xviii illustrates that the number of overweight children has been growing steadily over the past 40 years. Since 2001, the problem has been accelerating even faster.

## Back to the Bottom Line . . .

Do you find these statistics shocking? I do! With children spending most of their time being inactive, our school's population failing to meet minimum fitness standards, and our kids gaining weight, America is raising a generation of couch potatoes! And these bad habits are not something our children will simply "grow out of." Studies have shown that, as they age, children with a sedentary lifestyle will have a greater risk for obesity. Complications due to obesity include diseases and conditions such as hypertension, heart attacks, strokes, diabetes, and ulcers. Children who are unfit and overweight are more likely to have serious health issues when they are adults, such as high blood pressure, high cholesterol, Type 2 diabetes, stroke, heart attack—and more.

As parents, we need to find ways to promote activities that increase physical fitness and lead to healthier minds and bodies in our children.

Often, we may encourage unhealthy habits without realizing it. Again, ask yourself: what activities do you promote? Watching TV or running? Playing Nintendo or playing basketball?

---

2  *The Journal of the American Medical Association.* 2002; 288: 1728–1732.

The good news is: you can help guide your child to health and physical fitness.

This book will show you how.

## My Story . . .

I first became aware of my *own* children's lack of fitness when I noticed they were physically lagging behind their peers and were not scoring well on fitness tests. This was painfully embarrassing for me because, as a college professor, I was teaching future physical education teachers—yet at home I was failing to teach fitness to my own children! I became determined to write a plan to improve the level of fitness of our family. This book is based on that plan, and I have followed this program with my own children.

I have put years of knowledge and experience into this book—including the experiences that my wife and I shared with our children, as a family struggling to get fit.

## YOU MAY BE WONDERING . . .
## Can I Do It?

You may be thinking, "I want to do this, but do I have the knowledge, ability, and resources to make fitness and physical education activities part of my life with my children, right here at home? How much time will it take? How much preparation time will it require of me? How is my family going to manage all of this?"

You *can* do it! My wife and I have nine children, who we home-schooled, and we made physical activity a part of their schedule without taking time away from their core classes. This required *minimal* preparation time and very little expense.

## What Benefits Can I Expect?

The efforts you make now for your child will lead to a lifetime of good habits, since individuals who are physically active when they are young tend to continue to be active as adults.

And you will see immediate benefits, too. Children who are physically fit tend to have more energy, keep their body weight at a normal level, and are less likely to become sick. Plus, they sleep better (which means *you'll* sleep better, too!)

## My Story . . .

Children ages 3 to 6 typically have a lot of energy and want to be active and run. Our dining room has two doors, creating a circle between the kitchen and dining room. After the evening meal, our young children loved to run in circles, playing tag and making quite a bit of noise. This drove my wife and I crazy, as we were trying to relax and clean up after the meal.

What was the best solution for everyone? Rather than plant the children in front of the TV, we let them vent their natural energy, and sent them outside or downstairs to the basement where they could safely expend their energy and noise.

Allowing your children to release their natural energy, rather than force them to be still, will help your relationship with the child and encourage physical fitness.

You will also notice a change in your own level of fitness, too. I want to encourage parents to be role models by getting involved in their own fitness programs as well as family fitness activities.

Best of all, you will encourage family unity by enjoying physical activities together. Playing and exercising together will build memories of love for a lifetime.

## And Even Better . . .

Many studies have found a relationship between physical fitness and better academic performance. One experiment showed that public school children who exercised 80 minutes a week earned higher grades in language, math, natural science, and English than children who had no physical activity during the school day.

> **"Physical education programs** belong in elementary schools, not only because they promote health and well-being, but because they contribute tangibly to academic achievement. Researchers in France, Australia, Israel, and the United States have found that youngsters who partake in structured programs of vigorous exercise possess greater mental acuity and stronger interest in learning than those who do not."[3]

With your guidance, your children can develop habits that will keep them fit and healthy for a lifetime.

## HOW TO USE THIS BOOK

This book will give you the tools and knowledge to help you guide your children to a lifetime of physical fitness and weight control, with a minimum of equipment and expense. You will help

---

3   Ibid.

your children build the skills they need, and instill in them a desire to be fit.

Each section will teach you how to set up a personalized fitness program, tailor-made for each child.

Also included is a curriculum guide, with lesson plans and suggestions for effective games and activities that are also practical for the home.

## Who This Book is For

This book will help your children learn how to maintain a healthy body, and help them build sports skills. Older children can use this book like a textbook and read it on their own. However, this book is most effective when parents join the program.

This book is written for two specific types of families: one, for parents whose children attend school, and two, for families who home school their children. This guide has been used successfully by both types of families.

### PARENTS WHOSE CHILDREN ATTEND SCHOOL

If your children attend school, they are already enrolled in a physical education program. However, parents are also responsible for monitoring their child's level of fitness. I have created a parent guide for improving the fitness level of children using a variety of activities—many of which can be performed right at home on the weekends, after school, or during the summer.

### PARENTS WHO HOME SCHOOL THEIR CHILDREN

For home educating parents, I have provided curriculum guidelines and lesson plans in physical education, so parents who teach at home can

easily and successfully include physical education in their daily schedule.

**Home educators have** even more incentive to practice organized physical activity with the family. Forty-eight states have laws requiring that home schooled children receive physical education instruction from 20 to 60 minutes per week (recess does not count as instructional time).

Visit www.ncsl.org/programs/health/perequirement. html for a map detailing the requirements for each state, or call your state department of education.

### A NOTE FOR HOME SCHOOL FAMILIES . . .

There is a growing demand for states to follow California's model, and document their students' health and fitness level findings from annual fitness testing. Home schooling parents can start to meet these state requirements by following the recommendations in this book (planning activities for 20 minutes, three times a week, at a minimum).

I encourage home educators to add one component of physical education at a time so you do not feel overwhelmed. I suggest you start your child on a muscle-strengthening program as outlined in chapter 2. The next step is to have your child each day do one new game from chapter 4. Become familiar with the skills each game reinforces. You are then ready to use the lesson plans in chapter 6 and the labs in chapter 7. Aerobics in chapter 3 is usually the hardest for families, as it requires significant discipline, and therefore it should be started last.

## THE KEYS TO SUCCESS

I have compiled information and structured the physical activities in this book based on research from the following organizations:

♦ National Standards for Physical Education as set by The National Association for Sport and Physical Education (NASPE)
♦ Physical Education Model Content Standards for California Public Schools
♦ Canadian Association for Health, Physical Education, Recreation and Dance (CAHPERD)

Visit their web sites (listed at the back of the book) for more information. Regardless of how your children are educated—at home or at school—a good physical education program is key. The most successful programs include three key components: knowledge, fitness, and skills. Also, an added bonus: fun! Use this book to help your children become knowledgeable on how to maintain a healthy body, learn sport skills, and have fun while doing it.

### Knowledge

Children in junior high and senior high can use this book like a textbook. By reading the material and doing the labs, they can grow in their understanding of the functioning of the human body during exercise, and the relationship between exercise and good health. Parents can use this book as a teacher's lesson plan guide for all ages.

### Fitness

You can use this book to help you set up an appropriate exercise regimen. A muscular fitness plan is outlined in the chapter Muscular Strength, Endurance and Flexibility. If your child regularly participates in this plan (which takes approximately 40 minutes per week), they will be well on their way to meeting and exceeding the muscular strength standards set by the National Association for Sport and Physical Education (NASPE). Similarly, the Aerobic Fitness chapter outlines a cardiovascular fitness program that is a good start to meeting the NASPE's cardiovascular fitness standards for good health. This program will take 40 to 60 minutes each week.

### Skills

Sports are a great way to get fit—and have fun! The Lesson Plans chapter is written for elementary children, but much of the material will also apply to the upper grades. The Modified Games chapter contains games that can be done at home and are to be used with the lesson plans. The Labs chapter contains "hands on" experiments and activities that are designed to focus the learning on a fitness concept or a sport skill. The labs are designed so that little or no preparation is needed by the parent. By using these labs along with the lesson plans, any home educator should feel confident about teaching physical education.

### BONUS: FAMILY FUN!

Family games are a great way to have fun and shape up! The physical activities listed in this book can be used by any family, whether it is a home-schooling family or not. What is most important is that you build a healthy family and create good memories of having fun together as a family.

## YOU MAY BE WONDERING . . .

### Where Should I Exercise?

I have designed this book around the free spaces you have around you; bedroom, rec room, basement, garage, driveway, backyard and city park, etc. Just about any space you can think of will work!

### What Equipment Do I Need?

In the Appendix at the back of the book, I have listed equipment you will need. Much of the equipment includes basic items that you probably already have, such as a trash can, empty milk jugs, and socks. Other items are inexpensive and easy to find, such as beanbags, tennis balls, Nerf balls, and jump ropes. I encourage you to store all your sports equipment in one spot (large trash can or closet), so your children have quick and easy access to what they need.

### What if I Have One Child?

Many activities in this book can be done with only one child. If two players are required, you will become that playmate, or you can be creative and invite friends or neighbors to join in. Remember, your child will be more motivated if they can play with another child or a new friend, so make the effort to include other playmates.

### What if My Children are at Different Skill Levels?

In chapter 4 I have listed many different games to play along with "handicaps" with some of the games to make it easier for the younger child. Our whole family plays basketball lightning. Our "handicaps" are the younger you are, the closer you can be to the basket. With a little experience you can make creative "handicaps" for each of your children to make play more fair. Sometimes the children have more energy than I have. In that case I create handicaps so I do not have to run as much as they do.

### Get Started!

Tonight at dinner, start a discussion. You can begin by asking your child or children:

- Which is more important to you, academics or physical fitness?
- If you were to study academics less and exercise more, could you get better grades?
- Has the fitness of American children increased during the past 30 years?
- Do children imitate the habits of their parents in the areas of nutrition, exercise, and recreation?

### One Final Note . . .

I suggest you add physical education components slowly so you do not get overwhelmed. The order I recommend is as follows:

- First, start your child on the muscle-strengthening program as outlined in chapter 2. I recommend doing the exercises five days a week.
- Next, on a daily basis, have your children select one or two of the games listed in chapter 4. Continue playing one or two games every day, for two weeks. (It is important to be familiar with the skills each game reinforces before you begin the games.)

- You will then be ready to use the lesson plans in chapter 6 and the labs in chapter 7. Chapter 6 teaches a variety of body movement skills that are usually taught in elementary grades. Chapter 7 teaches specific sport skills that are taught in grades 7 to 12.

- The aerobics program in chapter 3 is usually the most challenging for families because it requires a good deal of discipline. I recommend trying this after you have mastered the other activities.

# Ways to Inspire Your Child

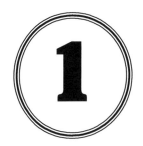

## YOU CAN BE AN INSPIRATION!

You may be thinking: how could I possibly inspire my child to get up off the couch, turn off the video game, and get fit?

### Remember . . .

You know your child better than any other person. You are in a unique position to influence, motivate, and shape your child's habits.

This chapter will give you creative ideas on how to get started.

## YOU CAN SET AN EXAMPLE

Have you ever wondered why many children will reach for a slice of pizza instead of an apple? In other words, have you ever wondered how children acquire likes and preferences? It's simple: What they see Mom or Dad do will mold their preferences and habits for life.

Our values and habits become those of our children. If they see you exercise, they will be inspired to imitate you and exercise, too. Studies have shown that parents who engage in an exercise program or sports, and who have a positive attitude toward fitness, motivate their children to engage in regular vigorous exercise, as well.[4]

## ASK YOUR CHILDREN TO JOIN YOU IN ACTIVITIES

If your children see that you are making time for exercise, then they will know it is important to you. Try having a special weekly family fitness event, such as walking, biking, or playing games. My wife has our older sons jog with her for her "protection," or the younger children ride their bikes while she jogs. She makes this time enjoyable so it has a positive imprint on our children's mind.

◇◇◇◇◇◇◇◇◇◇◇◇◇◇◇◇◇◇◇◇◇◇◇◇◇◇◇◇

**Parents of grade** school children who do no meaningful physical activity during the week:

**48%  Fathers**
**42%  Mothers**

—National Children and Youth Fitness Study

◇◇◇◇◇◇◇◇◇◇◇◇◇◇◇◇◇◇◇◇◇◇◇◇◇◇◇◇

## OTHER ROLE MODELS

To help motivate your children, you can introduce them to other healthy role models, too. But

---

4  *Research Quarterly for Exercise and Sport*, vol. 58, no. 4, 1987, p.323.

don't worry: you don't have to know a sports celebrity personally! There are plenty of great magazines, movies, and books about legendary athletes and world-famous teams available.

## Inspiring Films

There are many sports-related movies out there to choose from. Not all sport movies promote good character qualities. As a guide, I have listed some of my favorite films that are motivational and promote good character.

*Hoosiers* (1986) The true story of a small Indiana town that wins the state basketball tournament. (PG)

*Facing the Giants* (2006) A small-town football team wins the state title through hard work and teamwork. (G)

*Believe in Me* (2007) Based on a true story of a 1960s rural Oklahoma girls' basketball team that makes it to the state tournament against all odds. (PG)

*Pistol: The Birth of a Legend* (1991) The true story of basketball player Pete Maravich, who averaged an incredible 44.5 points per game in college. The film takes place during his eighth grade year of high school. He plays on the varsity basketball team but has to overcome difficult obstacles to become a starter. His father, a college basketball coach, teaches Pete discipline and dedication. (G)

*Chariots of Fire* (1981) The moving story of two young British sprinters competing during the 1924 Olympics. The running scenes in this film are unforgettable! (G)

*Brian's Song* (1971)  The biography of pro running back Brian Picallo, this is a story about friendship and overcoming barriers as well as achieving excellence in football. (G)

*Rocky* (1976)  Rocky is a very inspirational film, although the final fight scene may be too graphic for young viewers. Rocky is a small-time boxer who gets an opportunity to fight the heavyweight world champion. Rocky diligently trains physically and mentally for the fight. (PG)

*Mickey* (2004)  Mickey, a gifted 12-year-old boy, loves to play baseball. He cheats to make it to the Little League World Series. In the end the boy does the right thing and confesses his cheating. (PG)

*Ice Castles* (1978)  In this inspiring story, a gifted girl dreams of becoming a world class figure skater. A tragic accident blinds her, but she still trains as a figure skater.

*Ice Princess* (2005)  A 17-year-old girl presents a science project on the principles of physics in figure-skating. She becomes a figure skater in the process.

*Nadia* (1984)  The true story of the Rumanian gymnast, Nadia Comaneci, who scored a perfect 10 in the 1976 Olympics.

## Books

There are many inspirational biographies of sports stars. I think that the lives of the follow-ing sports legends are especially interesting and inspiring:

Pete Maravich (basketball)
Fran Tarkenton (football)
Reggie White (football)
Dennis Byrd (football)
Hank Aaron (baseball)
Jackie Robinson (baseball)
Michael Jordan (basketball)
Nancy Kerrigan (figure skating)
Carly Patterson (gymnastics)
Eric Liddehl (track)
Jim Ryan (track)
Jesse Owens (track)

Visit your local library or check out an on-line bookseller to find the latest titles on these sport greats. You can read the books with your child and discuss what kinds of challenges each individual faced, and how they overcame them.

## Magazines

My children enjoy:

**Sports Spectrum www.sportsspectrum.com**
Stories on current athletes (high school, college, pro) who are wholesome role models.

**Boy's Life www.boyslife.org**
Boy's Life usually carries a feature story on a child or young adult athlete.

**Sports Illustrated for Kids**
www.sikids.com
Similar to Sports Illustrated but focused on topics kids enjoy.

HOME SCHOOL FAMILY FITNESS

**Women's Sports Foundation www. womenssportsfoundation.org**

This web magazine is an educational organization dedicated to promoting girls and women in sports and fitness.

When the magazine arrives each month, set aside some time to sit down with your child and listen to what features they like most in the issue. Find ways to incorporate lessons or strategies from the articles into your exercise programs.

## REWARD THEIR ACCOMPLISHMENTS

Although the goal is to make fitness so fun that your kids enjoy it no matter what, keeping track of your child's progress and offering small rewards can be a great way to encourage them. Here are some things you can do:

* Keep track of personal records and use a gold star or a sticker when your child completes an activity.
* Once he or she reaches the assigned exercise goal, take him or her to a movie or let the child choose a family outing.
* Hide a small piece of sports equipment, such as a headband, water bottle, or keychain, at the end of a jogging path. Play the game "Hot and Cold" until your child finds the "treasure."
* Have an exercise party (kickball or soccer can be especially fun) and let your children invite their friends

**If you home school . . .**

Have the home school support group keep charts of families' aerobic points.

## HOST A "MINI-OLYMPICS!"

A day-long competition or a small challenge with family and friends can be good-spirited and fun.

In the family:

* Who can do the most sit-ups 30 days from now?
* Who can set the record for the most sit-ups this year?

Remember that the minimum number of sit-ups is different based on your child's age. Use the tables in chapter 5 to show the child age appropriate goals.

Include others:

* Have a kickball or soccer party with your children's friends.
* Help organize weekly or monthly neighborhood games.
* Invite two or three families to a Sunday afternoon soccer game in your yard.

## HAVE THEM TEACH OTHER CHILDREN

One of the best ways to learn something is to teach it to another person. Children feel grown up if they can teach what they know to others. Have them "play coach" and teach siblings or other families certain game-related skills, such as passing a football or trapping a soccer ball.

## EXPOSE THEM TO A VARIETY OF NEW ACTIVITIES

Encourage children to try new activities. Your child may discover an activity that he or she has a natural talent for or really enjoys. Also, meeting new friends with similar interests is a great motivator.

Try these resources:

♦ Community Education Services offer a variety of after school and Saturday classes for recreational activities such as learning to ride a unicycle, gymnastics, juggling, fencing, floor hockey, basketball, etc.

♦ Summer track and field meets are sponsored by universities, high schools, and clubs for ages 8 to adult.

♦ Sport camps—typically, day camps start at age 8 and resident camps start at age 10.

♦ Various organizations sponsor Bike-a-thons, Walk-a-thons, Jump-a-thons.

♦ Amateur Athletic Union sponsors a variety of youth sport activities.

**Discussion questions** for your child

• What book or video on sports would you like to check out of the library?

• What physical activity do you enjoy doing?

• What new activity would you like to try?

## FITNESS CONTRACT

Fitness experts say you are more likely to exercise consistently and meet your workout goals if you put it in writing and are held accountable by another person. Read the chapters on muscle-strengthening and aerobics to help you set realistic start points and goals. Then, fill out the contract below with your child.

**You could point** out to your child that sports stars sign contracts, too. And when they do, they have certain responsibilities to stick to, also!

# FITNESS CONTRACT

I, _____ (child's name) will
fulfill my goals in aerobic and muscle-strength fitness.

## Aerobic Fitness

My goal is to start at _____ aerobic fitness points the first week,
and improve 20 aerobic fitness points every following week. When I reach 300
aerobic points per week, I will maintain this level. I will accurately record my
points on the charts provided.

The activities I plan to do are:

_____

_____

## Muscle-Strength Fitness

I will do the following exercises the first week:

Sit-ups _____ Push-ups _____ Pull-ups _____ Kangaroo Jumps _____

The second week, I will add:

Sit-ups _____ Push-ups _____ Pull-ups _____ Kangaroo Jumps _____

## Schedule

The days I plan to exercise are:  **M   T   W   Th   F   Sa   Su**

The time of day I plan to exercise is: _____

## Parent's Responsibility

I will provide the following so that my child may fulfill this contract:

- the equipment needed
- the time needed
- transportation needed

I will also:

- remind my child of his above responsibilities
- remind my child to exercise once a day, at the particular time they have chosen and written down above
- monitor the progress of my child and give feedback when appropriate

♦ schedule special family fitness outings
♦ provide prompt rewards when they are earned

Other responsibilities: _____

## Child's Rewards

For outstanding accomplishments, my child can earn (circle which ones apply):

sleep-over with one friend
parent/child canoe ride
a day off from doing dishes
menu choice for one meal
permission to purchase a favorite item _____,
accessories for a hobby
choice of family outing
permission to have an exercise party (kickball, soccer party, etc.)
others _____

## Penalties For Not Fulfilling Contract

Child: (example: no desert for one night) _____

Parent: (example: doing the child's chore for one day, taking the garbage out)
_____

Date: _____

Signed and agreed upon by:

Child's signature: _____

Parent's signature: _____

**Remember . . .** you know your children better than anyone else, and you know the best way to inspire them. Find ways to encourage them to be physically active and make it fun for your children to be fit.

◇◇◇◇◇◇◇◇◇◇◇◇◇◇◇◇◇◇◇◇◇◇◇◇◇◇◇◇◇◇◇◇◇◇◇◇◇◇◇◇◇◇◇◇◇

**The goal is** to motivate your child to be fit—for a lifetime!

◇◇◇◇◇◇◇◇◇◇◇◇◇◇◇◇◇◇◇◇◇◇◇◇◇◇◇◇◇◇◇◇◇◇◇◇◇◇◇◇◇◇◇◇◇

# Muscular Strength, Endurance, and Flexibility

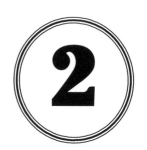

## BUILDING MUSCLE STRENGTH AND ENDURANCE

There is an old saying: "A journey of a thousand miles begins with one step." If you start your fitness program now and are consistent one day at a time, you will be able to reach your goal of physical fitness.

This chapter will explore good muscular health as it relates to strength, endurance, and flexibility of the muscles. It will give you a practical plan to help your children build healthy muscles at home with minimal expense and equipment.

### My story . . .

I found that my own children were lagging behind their peers in strength and sports skills. As a professional in physical education, I found this to be very embarrassing.

I sat down to figure out how I could motivate my children and assign them activities to do at home that would increase their physical fitness with a minimal amount of equipment. To start with, I assigned them four

> **An eagle builds** a nest one stick at a time, but when the nest is finished, it can weigh one ton!

callisthenic exercises to do, five days a week. I challenged them to improve each week and made an exercise diary to keep track of what they were doing.

How could I make sure they would do it? Their siblings tattled if they did not! And there is now a healthy competition among my children to have the top fitness record in the family.

## How Muscle Strength and Endurance is Developed

In order to be considered fit, an individual needs to build both muscle *strength* and *endurance*. *Muscle strength* is built by having a muscle move against resistance. Resistance can be provided by iron weights, rubber bands, body weight, or a fixed location, like a door frame.

When most people hear the phrase "muscle-strength training," they picture a muscular weight lifter, lifting barbells. This is called *heavy resistance strength training*, and it is often used to strengthen mature athletes for competition. However, heavy resistance strength training is potentially dangerous to young, preadolescent bodies and should not be used.

Muscle-strength training does not involve lifting massive amounts of very heavy weight. Instead, muscle-strength training, and the program I will outline here, strengthens the muscles gradually over time, and has many benefits, including:

- Strengthening the muscles around the joints provides protection from sprain, strain, and injury in sports or fitness activities.
- Strong muscles improve posture and protect the back from pain and injury.

- Children feel better about themselves when they are physically fit. All children like to feel "strong."
- Overall, strong muscles enable children to complete daily tasks more safely and efficiently. We are using our muscles all the time!

*Muscular endurance* is the ability to repeat an activity many times, or to hold a particular position for an extended amount of time. We exhibit endurance when doing activities such as:

- walking
- swimming
- playing tennis
- carrying a 1-year-old child on your hip for an hour

When you are exercising, you are building both muscle strength and endurance. Most exercises can emphasize endurance or strength depending how you perform it.

## Building Muscle Strength and Endurance Without Weights

To build both strength *and* endurance in children exercises should be done using light resistance with many repetitions. For example, instead of lifting a 5-pound weight 10 times, the child would lift a 2-pound weight 50 times.

However, the simplest and safest way to improve muscular strength and endurance is to do calisthenics. Calisthenics is a type of muscle training that uses your own body weight as resistance. It does not cost anything, and does not require any specialized equipment.

Examples of calisthenics are push-ups and chin-ups.

◇◇◇◇◇◇◇◇◇◇◇◇◇◇◇◇◇◇◇◇◇◇◇◇◇◇◇◇◇◇◇◇◇

**Strength Training is:**

1. Important
2. Doable
3. Fun
4. Inexpensive

◇◇◇◇◇◇◇◇◇◇◇◇◇◇◇◇◇◇◇◇◇◇◇◇◇◇◇◇◇◇◇◇◇

## UNDERSTANDING BONES AND MUSCLES OF THE HUMAN BODY

In order to exercise properly, it is important to understand how bones and muscles work together.

## Major Bones of the Body

Man is a vertebrate and has an endoskeleton (internal skeleton) for support. A normal adult has 206 bones. The bones are like the poles of a camping tent; bones support the body the way tent poles support the fabric of the tent. Softer tissues actually attach to the bones for support.

The bones serve three major purposes in the following ways:

♦ make red blood cells
♦ provide anchors for the muscles and facilitate movement
♦ provide protection for parts of the body (for example, the skull protects the brain, and the ribs protect the heart and lungs)

## Joints

The meeting place of two bones is called an articulation, known as a joint. There are three types of joints, defined by the amount of movement the joint allows:

1. Synarthrodial—The joint that allows no movement. Example: Skull
2. Amphiarthrodial—The joint that moves slightly. Example: Spine
3. Diathrodial—The joint that allows free movement. Examples: Hinge Joint—Finger; Ball and Socket Joint—Shoulder

## Major Muscles of the Body

There are over 600 muscles in the body. These muscles make up half of our body weight. Muscles are attached to the bones and move the bones by pulling. The muscle is like a rope: it can only pull on the bone, not push it. When we bend our elbow or use the set of muscles around a joint, we are able to move the arm up and down because there are two sets of muscles: one muscle to pull the bone up, and another muscle to pull the bone down. The arm bends up at the elbow by the bicep muscle, and moves back down by the triceps muscle.

There are three kinds of muscles:

♦ Voluntary (the brain can control the movement) Example: biceps moving the arm
♦ Involuntary (the brain cannot control the movement) Example: intestines
♦ Cardiac Example: heart

## UNDERSTANDING ISOMETRIC AND ISOTONIC EXERCISE

It is important to understand the difference between these two key types of exercise before you begin a program to build muscle strength and endurance. This way, you have an understanding of how your joints and muscles interact.

# Major Bones of the Body

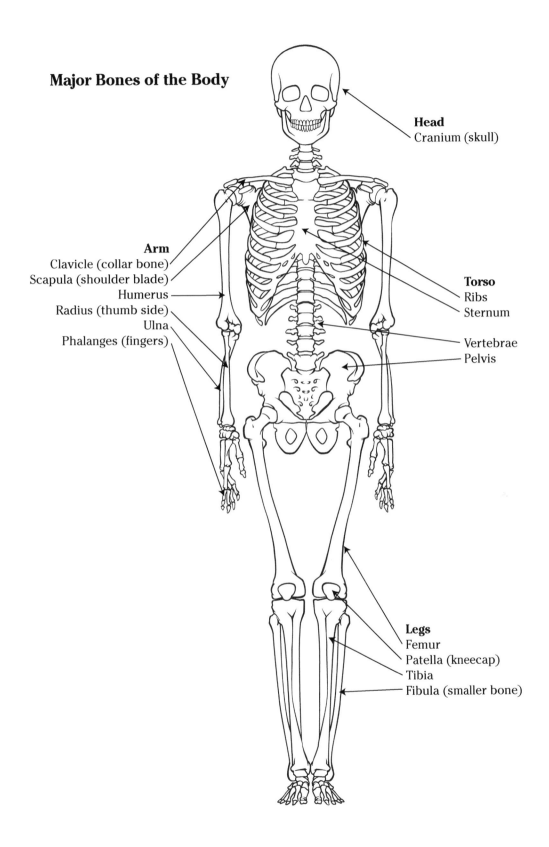

**Head**
Cranium (skull)

**Arm**
Clavicle (collar bone)
Scapula (shoulder blade)
Humerus
Radius (thumb side)
Ulna
Phalanges (fingers)

**Torso**
Ribs
Sternum

Vertebrae
Pelvis

**Legs**
Femur
Patella (kneecap)
Tibia
Fibula (smaller bone)

MUSCULAR STRENGTH, ENDURANCE, AND FLEXIBILITY

## Major Visible Muscles of Man, Ventral (front) Side

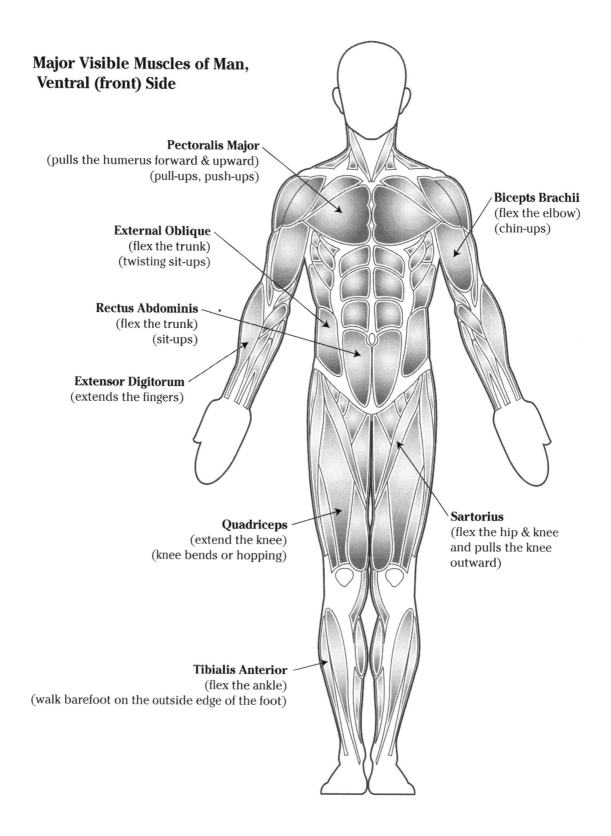

**Pectoralis Major**
(pulls the humerus forward & upward)
(pull-ups, push-ups)

**Biceps Brachii**
(flex the elbow)
(chin-ups)

**External Oblique**
(flex the trunk)
(twisting sit-ups)

**Rectus Abdominis**
(flex the trunk)
(sit-ups)

**Extensor Digitorum**
(extends the fingers)

**Quadriceps**
(extend the knee)
(knee bends or hopping)

**Sartorius**
(flex the hip & knee
and pulls the knee
outward)

**Tibialis Anterior**
(flex the ankle)
(walk barefoot on the outside edge of the foot)

# Major Visible Skeletal Muscles of Man, Dorsal (rear) Side

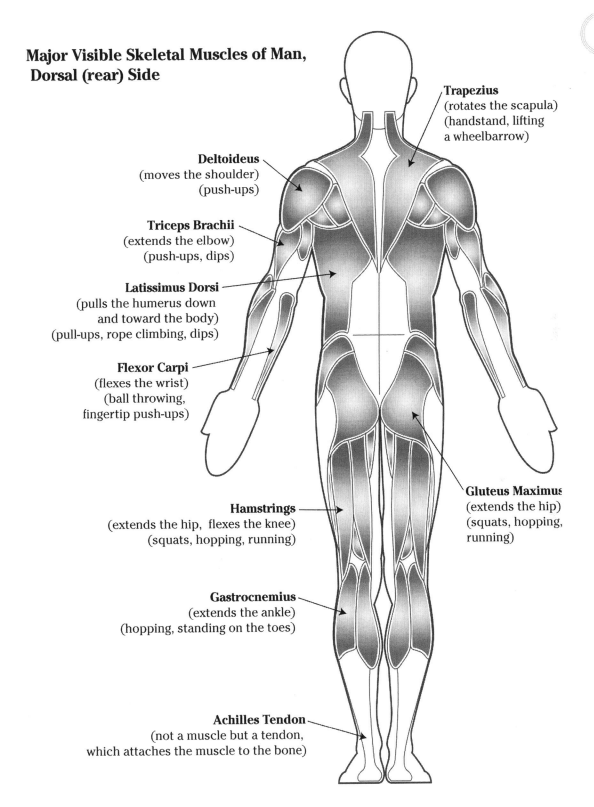

**Trapezius**
(rotates the scapula)
(handstand, lifting
a wheelbarrow)

**Deltoideus**
(moves the shoulder)
(push-ups)

**Triceps Brachii**
(extends the elbow)
(push-ups, dips)

**Latissimus Dorsi**
(pulls the humerus down
and toward the body)
(pull-ups, rope climbing, dips)

**Flexor Carpi**
(flexes the wrist)
(ball throwing,
fingertip push-ups)

**Gluteus Maximus**
(extends the hip)
(squats, hopping,
running)

**Hamstrings**
(extends the hip, flexes the knee)
(squats, hopping, running)

**Gastrocnemius**
(extends the ankle)
(hopping, standing on the toes)

**Achilles Tendon**
(not a muscle but a tendon,
which attaches the muscle to the bone)

## What is Isometric Exercise?

Isometric exercise is a type of strength training where the angle of the joint does not change during the exercise. If your child stands in a doorway and pushes with her hands against the door frame, the muscles work but the elbow and shoulder joints do not move. Isometric exercises are primarily used for medical rehabilitation purposes but can easily be incorporated into any exercise program for children. Straight Leg Raises (listed in this chapter) is an example of isometric exercise.

## What is Isotonic Exercise?

In an isotonic exercise the contracting muscle shortens, the joint moves, and the angle changes. This takes place when you pick up a glass of water and bring it to your lips. The shoulder and elbow joints move and the joint angles change.

Isotonic exercise can be done with or without equipment such as free weights, barbells, or fixed equipment like a Nautilus machine, or can be done with just your body weight, such as a chin-up and push-up.

**A caution:** As I mentioned earlier, the use of weight-lifting equipment to build muscle strength in elementary children is usually not recommended, unless it is for physical therapy purposes. The child's bone growth plates could be injured by lifting very heavy weights. If children are actively playing and running about, doing calisthenics, they will develop normally without using weight-lifting equipment. I do not recommend using weight-lifting equipment regularly until approximately ninth grade in order to reduce potential injuries, and then only with close supervision and instruction.

Below, I have included several exercises for your children that build both muscle strength and endurance. I begin with isotonic exercises, and then list some isometric exercises.

## ISOTONIC EXERCISES FOR THE UPPER AND LOWER BODY THAT BUILD STRENGTH AND ENDURANCE

### Sit-Up: Abdominal Strength & Endurance

**Muscles Developed:** Abdominal muscles (rectus abdominis, obliquus abdomini internus and externus) and hip flexor muscles (psoas major and iliacus)

Lower back pain is a common problem in the USA. Weak abdominal and back muscles contribute to this problem. Sit-ups help strengthen some of the muscles that are needed for good posture.

**Description:** Begin by laying flat on the floor. Knees should be bent at least 90 degrees, and feet should be flat on the floor. Hands should be crossed over the chest, hugging the opposite shoulders. Tuck the chin into the chest, and raise the shoulder blades off the floor. Continue to curl the upper body until the wrists touch the knees. Lower back down until the shoulder blades are just off the ground.

- Alternate touching the right wrist to the left knee and the left wrist to the right knee.
- As many sit-ups as possible should be completed before stopping. Doing these exercises *slowly* is more beneficial than doing them quickly.

**A caution:** You may have seen some versions of the sit-up where the individual puts their hands behind their neck. Putting the hands behind the neck during sit-ups can cause neck injuries from

## 1. Push up on box/stool

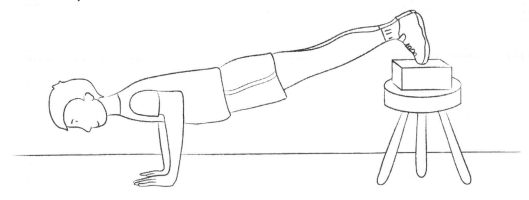

excessive jerking on the head with the hands. So be sure to place hands on opposite shoulders, as detailed in the instructions above.

◇◇◇◇◇◇◇◇◇◇◇◇◇◇◇◇◇◇◇◇◇◇◇◇◇◇◇◇◇◇

**Be sure to** breathe! It is not good to hold your breath during exercise, because it can raise blood pressure.

◇◇◇◇◇◇◇◇◇◇◇◇◇◇◇◇◇◇◇◇◇◇◇◇◇◇◇◇◇◇

## The Crunch

One variation of the sit-up that is good for individuals prone to lower back pain is called a crunch. In a crunch sit-up, only the shoulders are lifted off the floor, so that only the abdominal muscles do the work. (In a full sit-up, both the abdominal and hip flexor muscles are worked).

## Push-Up: Upper Body Strength & Endurance

**Muscles Developed:** arms (triceps), shoulder (deltoid), trunk (pectoralis major, erector spinae, abdominals)

**Description:** Begin with the hands on the floor, under the shoulders. The fingers should point forward. The toes are tucked under, gripping the floor. Extend the elbows and raise the entire body off the floor until the elbows are straight. Keep the back as straight as possible. Bend the elbows and slowly lower the body until only the chin touches the floor. Raise back up and do as many push-ups as possible.

**Hint:** if the feet tend to slide, put the feet against a wall.

**Variation for weaker individuals:** Some individuals may not have the upper body strength to do a regular push-up. They can do a modified push-up, raising up from the knees rather than from the toes.

**Variations for advanced individuals:** To challenge the stronger individual, try these variations.

- ◆ **Clap push-up.** Push up vigorously and clap the hands together before returning the hands to the floor.
- ◆ **Rocky push-ups** Put one hand behind your back. Do push- ups with one arm.
- ◆ **Box push-ups** Put your feet on a box one foot off the ground.

## Pull-Up: Upper Body Strength and Endurance

**Muscles Developed:** arms (biceps, brachioradialis), upper chest and back (trapezius and latissimus dorsi)

**Equipment:** You will need simple equipment that can support your child's weight for this exercise. A swing set frame can work, or a wooden or iron bar hung in the garage or basement. (Caution: if you install a bar yourself, make sure it is secured properly. Test the bar to make sure it can hold the weight of an adult, so you can be sure your child will not break the bar.)

**Description:** Grip the bar so that the feet are off the ground. Pull up until the chin is above the bar. Lower back down slowly, to the starting position.

**Note:** if your child is not able to do a full pull-up, she should simply pull herself up as far as she can—this will still build strength.

**Hint:** Begin with palms facing in. As your child becomes stronger, she should try it with palms facing out.

## Isometric Chin-up

If your child cannot lift her body and complete one single chin-up, have her start with isometric chin-ups, instead of an isotonic exercise.

The child should hang with elbows bent, holding the normal chin-up position for as long as possible.

**Note:** My children love to do pull-ups on the door frames of our house. If your child is going to do this, make sure the door frames are properly secured first!

## Kangaroo Jumps: Lower Body Strength and Endurance

**Muscles Developed:** Calf (gastrocnemius), knee extensors (quadriceps), hip extensors (hamstrings, gluteus maximus)

**Description:** Start in a standing position with the right foot in front of the left. Bend the knees to a 90-degree angle. Bend at the waist until the

upper part of the body is bent at a 45-degree angle. The arms should hang straight down, with the wrists approximately at the height of the knees. Extend the knees and jump as high as possible. While in the air, switch the feet so the left foot is in front of the right foot. Land and repeat. Do as many as possible.

**Caution:** For some children, bending the knee more than 90 degrees may put too much stress on the knees and cause pain. If your child develops knee pain, stop doing this exercise until pain is gone. When you resume, make sure that the knees do not bend more than 90 degrees.

If your child has sore knees, have her start with the isometric squats, instead of an isotonic exercise.

## Isometric Squats

**Description:** Place the back against a wall and lower the body until the thighs are parallel to the floor. Shuffle the feet until your lower legs are parallel to the wall. The knees should be bent to a 90-degree angle. Extend the arms in front of the body, and hold the position for 10 to 30 seconds. Repeat 2 to 3 times.

## ISOMETRIC EXERCISES FOR THE UPPER & LOWER BODY THAT BUILD STRENGTH AND ENDURANCE

These exercises build strength and endurance without putting stress on the joints.

## Flying: Back Strength and Endurance

**Muscles Developed:** Back (erector spinae), hip extensors (gluteus maximus), shoulder girdle

## 2. Flying in flat position

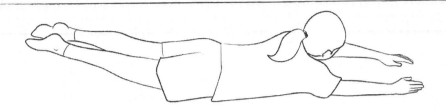

(rhomboid, trapezius), shoulder external rotators (deltoid, teres minor)

**Description:** Lie face-down on the floor. Place the arms in front of the head. Raise the arms, head, and chest as well as thighs and feet off the floor (everything except the tummy). The shoulders and collar bone should between one and two inches off the floor. Hold the position for 10 to 30 seconds and repeat 2 to 3 times.

## Shoulder Exercise

**Muscles Developed:** shoulder (deltoid)

**Description:** Stand in a doorway with hands at the sides and palms facing the thighs. Raise hands up and out against the door frame. Hold for 10 to 20 seconds and repeat 2 to 3 times.

## Leg Extensions

**Muscles Developed:** thigh (quadracept)

**Description:** Stand next to the side of a bed (should be about 18 inches high). Face away from the bed with the backs of the legs against the bed. Bend the right leg and lift it to rest on the bed. The right leg should be bent at about a 90-degree angle. The left leg is straight and stands firmly on the floor. Push the right leg into the bed as forcefully as possible and hold for 10 to 30 seconds. Repeat 2 to 3 times and change legs. Remember to breathe!

## Calf Raises

**Muscles Developed:** calf (gastrocnemius)

**Description:** Stand next to a sturdy chair (or any fixed object) and hold onto it for balance. Stand on the right leg and raise the left leg into the air. Bend the left knee and rest the left foot on the back of the right calf. Lift up the right leg and come to stand on the toes. Hold the position for 10 to 30 seconds and repeat 2 to 3 times. Then repeat for the left leg.

**Don't give up!** After following this program, my children met with great success. My 8-year-old set a personal push-up record of 320 push-ups in 20 minutes (Later, as a teenager, he could walk on his hands!) My 10-year-old set a personal record of 410 sit-ups in 20 minutes. Both of them started at 4 push-ups and 10 sit-ups, respectively!

All of my children have improved their physical fitness, and have had fun doing it. They feel good about having healthy exercise habits and they love being "strong." Hopefully, I am helping them to establish a lifelong love for healthy exercise.

HOME SCHOOL FAMILY FITNESS

## SPECIALIZED STRENGTH AND ENDURANCE EXERCISES

The purpose of the previous exercises is to develop general body strength. This next section suggests exercises that can be done to help prevent injuries common in specific sports, or to strengthen an injured muscle.

A general rule of thumb is not to do isotonic exercises (the joint moves as the muscle contracts) if the exercise causes pain. Instead, isometric exercises (the joint does not move as muscle contracts) should be used to strengthen injured joints. For this reason, many of the exercises below are isometric.

**Please note:** When your child is seriously injured, be sure to consult the proper medical personnel. They will make sure that the correct rehabilitative exercises are performed.

## Shoulder Injury Prevention

The most common baseball injury is to the rotator cuff in the shoulder. In April, players everywhere get "baseball fever" when the weather turns warm. They rush outside to play catch—often after spending months indoors. All this hard throwing, after 9 months of inactivity, often causes shoulder strain and injury.

Only light throwing should be done for the first 2 weeks, and exercises for the throwing muscles should be done 2 months before the season starts. Here are two good exercises to strengthen the throwing shoulder 2 months before baseball season starts. Of course, these exercises can be practiced indoors during winter weather.

## Pre-Throwing Exercise: Shoulder Strength & Endurance

3. Pre-throwing exercise

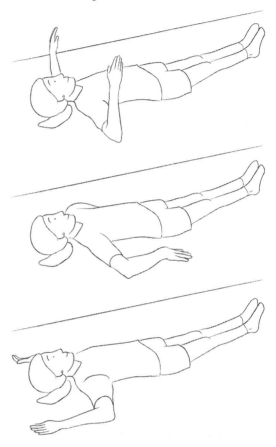

**Muscles Developed:** Rotator cuff, inward rotators (teres major, subscapularis, deltoid, latisimus dorsi)

**Description:** Begin lying face-up on the floor, with the elbows bent at a 90-degree angle and the palms facing the ceiling. Raise both hands up, while keeping the elbows on the floor. (Both arms up will resemble goal posts). Complete three sets of 35 repetitions. Start with no weight in the hands, and, if the full 105 repetitions can be completed without difficulty, add a half-pound weight the next day (a pair of small pliers or can of tuna can be used if a weight is not available). Continue to add weight at a consistent rate, up to 5 pounds.

## Pre-Throwing Exercise 2: Shoulder Strength & Endurance

**Muscles Developed:** Rotator cuff, outward rotators (deltoid, infraspinatus, teres minor)

**Description:** Set up a chair so that the side is parallel to the edge of the table. Sit down and stack phone books under the elbow until the shoulder is level with the elbow. Elbow should stay bent at a 90-degree angle throughout the exercises. Begin with hand on the surface of the table, with palm facing down. Raise the hand straight up and back, keeping the elbow bent. Complete three sets of 35 repetitions. Start with no weight in the hands, and, if the full 105 repetitions can be completed without difficulty, add a half-pound weight the next day.

## Knee Injury Prevention
### STRAIGHT LEG RAISES: KNEE STRENGTH & ENDURANCE

In sports, the knee is very susceptible to injury. Young basketball players can twist the knee while pivoting, and 12- to 15-year-old girls, who may not have built up all of their muscle strength, are especially prone to injuring the knee in sports such as volleyball. You can help your child prevent these twists and sprains of the knee by strengthening the knee muscles. The leg extension exercises described below will strengthen the knee without aggravating the joint.

**Muscles Developed:** Knee extensors (quadriceps)

**Description:** Begin by lying on the floor, face up, with left knee bent. Keep the right leg straight. Tighten the right quadricep and raise the right heel off the floor. Be sure to keep the knee straight. Hold this position for 10 seconds. Then return to the rest position and rest for 5 seconds. Repeat this exercise 10 times, then repeat with the left leg. Every day, increase by one repetition until 3 sets of 30 repetitions can be completed.

As the legs get stronger, weights can be added. Weights can be created by putting objects in two socks, and tying the socks together at the top. Canned food, small tools, rocks, or nuts and bolts make good weights. Do 3 sets of 30 repetitions before adding weights.

## Ankle Injury Prevention
### ANKLE ALPHABET: ANKLE STRENGTH & ENDURANCE

Shin splints is a common injury in sports that involve running on a hard surface (such as basketball and tennis). A shin split causes pain in the front part of the lower leg or occasionally in the calf. Strengthening the muscles of the ankle is the best prevention for this injury.

**Muscles Developed:** Ankle (gastrocnemius, soleus, tibialis anterior and posterior, extensor digitorium, peroneus, flexor digitorum)

**Description:** Spell the alphabet with your foot by pretending you have a pencil in your toes. Make big letters.

### ANKLE WALK

Ankle sprains are common in sports involving running and jumping (skating, basketball, gymnastics). Ankles can be strengthened and sprains prevented by walking alternately on the inside, outside, toes, and heels of the feet. Note: Walking on the heels and toes will also help prevent shin splints.

**Muscles Developed:** Ankle (tibialis, anterior extensor digitorum)

**Description:** Walk 15 feet each in the following manner: on the inside of your foot, outside of your foot, heel, and toes.

## FLEXIBILITY

Have you ever observed a baby lift his leg up to his head and put a toe in his mouth? It is hard to imagine an adult doing the same! Children are naturally flexible, but, from my experience, this flexibility diminishes with age for both boys and girls. This is why, around the age of 8 or 9, stretching exercises should be introduced to help maintain flexibility.

**Flexibility is also** really important for adults. Although they may not know it, many adults who experience lower back pain may be suffering as a result of lack of flexibility in the hamstring muscle. The lower back pain can subside when the person restores flexibility to the hamstring muscles.

As I mentioned in the Introduction, flexibility is one of the key elements of fitness. Flexibility contributes to a healthy body by helping to prevent joint injuries and pain. Light stretching should be done as part of the warm up activity before starting strenuous exercise. Flexibility exercises should be done slowly, with no bouncing, and never beyond the point of mild discomfort. Below are several recommended stretches.

## Sit and Reach Stretch

**Muscles Stretched:** Hip adductors and extensors (hamstrings), lower back muscles (erector spinae)

**Description:** Sit on the floor with legs spread apart. Gradually reach forward as far as possible. Hold this position for 5 seconds, then return to the starting position. Do one set of 10 repetitions.

## Calf Stretch

The calf should be stretched before and after running to prevent muscle stiffness and soreness.

4. Stretching calf against wall

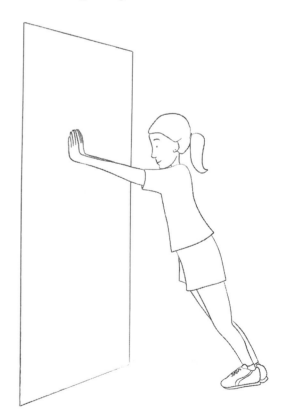

**Muscles Stretched:** Calf (gastrocnemius), shoulder adductors (pectoralis)

**Description:** Stand at arm's length from a wall or corner. Place hands slightly higher and slightly wider than your shoulders. Lean forward, bend your arms slightly, and slowly lower your face towards the wall. Keep your back and knees straight. Hold the stretch for 30 seconds. Straighten your arms and push your body back to the starting point. Repeat this exercise four to five times.

## Camel and Cat Stretch

Lower back pain is common in sports. This exercise can help reduce or prevent back pain.

**Muscles Stretched:** Back (erector spinae)

**Description:** Position yourself on your hands and knees. Arch your back as high as possible and hold the position for 5 seconds. Lower your back as low as possible and hold the position for 5 seconds. Do one set of 10 repetitions.

## EXERCISE PLAN

As I pointed out in chapter 1, making exercise a part of the family routine is very important. Here are some tips to make exercise a part of your family life.

## Have equipment

Simple backyard equipment can make exercise fun! Secure rope to a tree branch to encourage climbing, which will build upper body strength. If you don't have adequate room in your yard, make use of the play sets at a local park.

**Note:** Be sure any equipment in your back yard is set up properly to support your child's body weight. Before securing anything with knots, be certain your knots are properly tied and strong.

## Plan a monthly family outing

Visit the local playground and play on the jungle gym. Find a nature preserve in your area and go hiking, canoeing, or bicycling.

## Have a monthly family contest

Test all the family members for their personal best in several activities and then re-test every month for improvement, Mom and Dad included!

Keep a record book of personal bests for each member in the family.

## Have the home school support group give monthly awards

- ◆ Give awards to those who improve.
- ◆ Give awards for those who are consistent.
- ◆ Keep a record for each age group and display it (most sit-ups, etc.).

## Meet with another family

The families can find ways to exercise together. For example, invite two or three families for a Sunday afternoon kickball game.

## Neighborhood records

Keep an informal record book for children in the neighborhood (most sit-ups, etc.).

## Write a contract with your child

Setting and reaching goals can be a very powerful motivator. See chapter—(page ) for instructions on how to create a fitness contract.

## Monitoring Improvement

It is also important to schedule an exercise plan, and to keep records of your child's improvement.

Daily records should be kept by each child. Written records allow the child to see his improvement and give the parent a way to monitor the consistency and amount of exercise. Have the child write the number of repetitions he did for each exercise on the Muscle Strength & Endurance Log (see end of chapter.)

The layout of the log allows the parent to easily see the improvement of the children through the weeks and also reveals the days they miss their exercises.

Save the completed log sheets because it is motivating for a child to look at logs from past months and see evidence of their improvement.

For added motivation, we give our children a reward of a morning snack after they have completed their exercises.

## Assigning Excersises

You should assign exercises in two categories: muscle strength and endurance, and flexibility. Assign specialized exercises based on your child's needs.

### STRENGTH AND ENDURANCE

Assign *sit-ups, push-ups, pull-ups, kangaroo jumps, and flying* five days a week. These five exercises will work the major muscle groups of the body. The specialized exercises can be added when appropriate.

It will take 10 to 15 minutes to complete the exercises. A reasonable goal is to improve by one sit-up, push-up, kangaroo jump, etc., each week.

**Note:** most children will probably improve their performance in pull-ups at a slower rate than in the other exercises.

### FLEXIBILITY

Assign the stretching exercises three to five times a week starting at the age of 8 or 9 (limited flexibility usually does not become a problem with children until age 8 or 9).

◇◇◇◇◇◇◇◇◇◇◇◇◇◇◇◇◇◇◇◇◇◇◇◇◇◇◇◇◇◇◇◇

**What is the Best Time to Exercise?**

For home-educated children, mid-morning is a good time to do exercises; it lets the little wiggles come out after sitting and doing book work (after exercising, children will be more ready to sit quietly).

Exercising with Dad before or after the evening meal is also a good time for children to exercise—and spend time with Dad!

◇◇◇◇◇◇◇◇◇◇◇◇◇◇◇◇◇◇◇◇◇◇◇◇◇◇◇◇◇◇◇◇

# Muscle Strength and Endurance Log

Have your child record the repetitions he does for each exercise on a daily basis.

Month _____

| SUNDAY | MONDAY | TUESDAY | WEDNESDAY | THURSDAY | FRIDAY | SATURDAY |
|---|---|---|---|---|---|---|
| S | S | S | S | S | S | S |
| Push | Push | Push | Push | Push | Push | Push |
| Pull | Pull | Pull | Pull | Pull | Pull | Pull |
| K | K | K | K | K | K | K |
| F | F | F | F | F | F | F |
| S | S | S | S | S | S | S |
| S | S | S | S | S | S | S |
| Push | Push | Push | Push | Push | Push | Push |
| Pull | Pull | Pull | Pull | Pull | Pull | Pull |
| K | K | K | K | K | K | K |
| F | F | F | F | F | F | F |
| S | S | S | S | S | S | S |
| S | S | S | S | S | S | S |
| Push | Push | Push | Push | Push | Push | Push |
| Pull | Pull | Pull | Pull | Pull | Pull | Pull |
| K | K | K | K | K | K | K |
| F | F | F | F | F | F | F |
| S | S | S | S | S | S | S |
| S | S | S | S | S | S | S |
| Push | Push | Push | Push | Push | Push | Push |
| Pull | Pull | Pull | Pull | Pull | Pull | Pull |
| K | K | K | K | K | K | K |
| F | F | F | F | F | F | F |
| S | S | S | S | S | S | S |
| S | S | S | S | S | S | S |
| Push | Push | Push | Push | Push | Push | Push |
| Pull | Pull | Pull | Pull | Pull | Pull | Pull |
| K | K | K | K | K | K | K |
| F | F | F | F | F | F | F |
| S | S | S | S | S | S | S |

* S = Sit-up, Push = Push-up, Pull = Pull-up, K = Kangaroo Jump, F = Flying

## TEST WHAT YOU KNOW

First, have your child memorize the major bones
and muscles. Then, assign the following quizzes.

## Major Visible Muscles of Man, Ventral (front) Side

Write the names of the muscles.

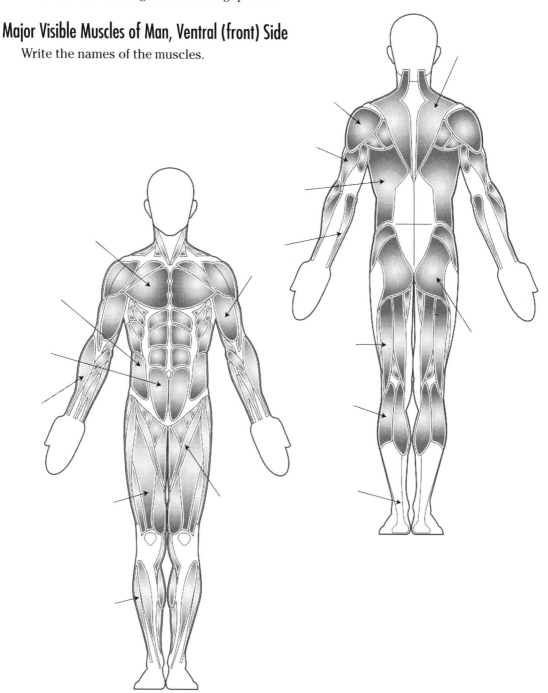

MUSCULAR STRENGTH, ENDURANCE, AND FLEXIBILITY

# Major Bones Test

Write the names of the bones.

**Major Bones of the Body**

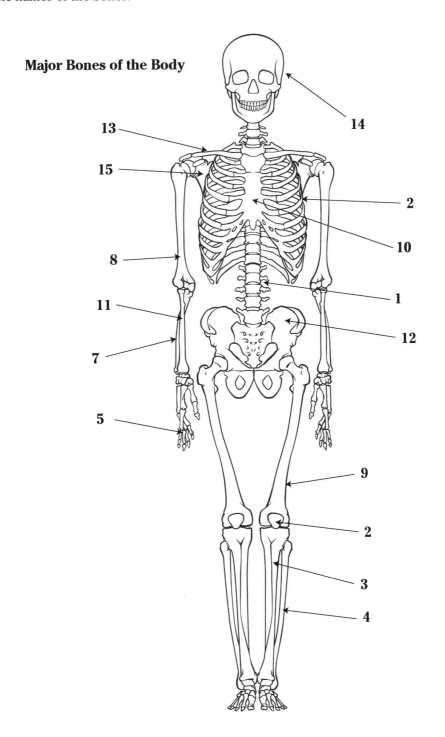

MUSCULAR STRENGTH, ENDURANCE, AND FLEXIBILITY

## Major Bones Test Answers

1. Spine or Vertebrae
2. Ribs
3. Tibia
4. Fibula
5. Phalanges
6. Patella
7. Ulna
8. Humerus
9. Femur
10. Sternum
11. Radius
12. Pelvis
13. Clavicle
14. Cranium
15. Scapula

## Questions to be completed by the child

A sit-up develops which muscles?

A push-up develops which muscles?

A pull-up develops what muscle?

A kangaroo jump develops what muscle?

What stretching exercise will increase flexibility of the hamstring muscles?

Name the three types of joints.

Name the three types of muscles.

## Review the following Key Terms with your child

**Muscle Strength**—The amount of force that can be exerted by a muscle group for one movement or repetition.

**Muscle Endurance**—The ability of a muscle group to maintain a continuous contraction or repetition over a period of time.

**Muscle Soreness**—Muscle pain resulting in possible chemical (lactic acid buildup) or physical changes in the muscle tissue.

**Overload**—Forcing a muscle to contract at a maximum or near maximum tension.

**Isometric Exercise**—A contraction performed against a fixed or immovable resistance, where tension is developed in the muscle but there is no movement in the joint.

**Circuit Training**—A combination of strength and endurance exercises performed in sequence.

# Aerobic Fitness

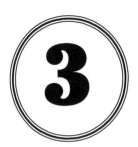

## WHAT IS AEROBIC FITNESS?

In the previous chapter, I outlined ways in which you can help your children build strong muscles. In fact, as we use our muscles over a period of time, building their strength and endurance, we are also engaging in something called *aerobic fitness*.

Aerobic fitness is defined by two key components:
1. the ability of all parts of the body (heart, lungs, arteries, veins, and blood) to work together to deliver fuel (oxygen and nutrients) to the muscle cells
2. the ability of those muscle cells to use that fuel (oxygen and nutrients) most efficiently

◇◇◇◇◇◇◇◇◇◇◇◇◇◇◇◇

**Parents are always** asking me, "How much exercise is enough for my child?" This chapter answers that question.

◇◇◇◇◇◇◇◇◇◇◇◇◇◇◇◇

## HOW DOES IT WORK?

Aerobic fitness plays an important role in the way our body works, every day.

With every breath we take, we are delivering valuable oxygen to our bodies. Oxygen is taken in through the lungs and passed onto the red blood cells. The newly-oxegenated red blood cells travel throughout the body through the bloodstream, which is pumped through the circulatory system by the powerful muscle of the heart. In this way, all the organs and cells in the body receive the oxygen they need.

Why is oxygen so important? For one, cells use oxygen to convert nutrients (carbohydrates and fats) into energy.

When we exercise, sprint for the bus, or do anything that raises our heart rate, our body requires that the cells manufacture a greater amount of energy. This means that the cells demand more oxygen—and fast. The lungs, heart, and blood vessels have to work extra hard to deliver that oxygen all throughout the body.

When the cells' demand for oxygen exceeds the body's ability to deliver it, fatigue sets in. We become fatigued because our body is no longer able to continue at the same intensity level—so the system must slow down, or stop altogether.

◇◇◇◇◇◇◇◇◇◇◇◇◇◇◇◇◇◇◇◇◇◇◇◇◇◇◇◇◇◇◇◇

**A person with** a high level of aerobic fitness has an increased ability to deliver and utilize the fuel (oxygen and nutrients) efficiently.

◇◇◇◇◇◇◇◇◇◇◇◇◇◇◇◇◇◇◇◇◇◇◇◇◇◇◇◇◇◇◇◇

Let's look inside the body and learn more about what happens when a person increases his or her aerobic fitness level through aerobic exercise. Here are a few of the changes that take place:

- ◆ The heart muscle is like any other muscle, and increases in size and strength as it is trained. A stronger heart has the ability to pump more blood with each heartbeat.
- ◆ More tiny blood vessels (capillaries) are created. The increased number of blood vessels allows faster delivery of oxygen to the cells.
- ◆ The red blood cell count increases so the blood has the ability to carry more oxygen.
- ◆ The size and number of mitochondria in each cell, and their ability to burn fat, increases. (The mitochondria are responsible for producing the energy needed in each cell.)

## BENEFITS OF AEROBIC EXERCISE
### Reduces the Risk of Many Diseases

Approximately 50 percent of all deaths in the United States are related to coronary heart diseases. Experts agree that regular aerobic exercise will greatly reduce the risk of coronary heart disease, strokes, diabetes, high blood pressure, ulcers, and other diseases.

### Maintains Proper Body Weight

Aerobic exercise burns calories and may increase the basic metabolic rate, which can help people lose weight and make it easier for people to maintain their desired body weight. As we examined in the Introduction, the number of American children ages 6 to 11 who are overweight is rising at an alarming rate—be reminded, from 1963 to 2000 the number increased 400%!

Besides being unhealthy for children when they are young, kids who are overweight are more likely to be overweight as adults. Helping children maintain their proper body weight through aerobic exercise will help them be healthy, and ensure that they do not become overweight as they age.

## Creates Stronger Bones

Aerobic exercise increases bone density, which makes bones stronger and less likely to break.

## Increased Intellectual Capacity

Research studies in Australia, France, Israel, and the United States have found that school-age children who participate in regular vigorous aerobic exercise get better grades and have a stronger interest in learning than those who do not do exercise.[5,6] Couldn't we all benefit from increasing our mental edge?

## HOW TO TRAIN THE BODY AEROBICALLY

Aerobic training begins when the body is challenged to perform physically. Then, the process begins that, over time, will strengthen muscles and improve performance of organs. Just as the biceps are strengthened by lifting a weight, the heart is strengthened when it has to work hard.

I have divided aerobic training into four components. These are the four key ways in which

---

5  The Journal of the American Medical Association. 2002; 288: 1728–1732
6  "First Lessons: A Report on Elementary Education in America," by the U.S. Department of Education, 1986

we must exercise in order to train ourselves effectively.

- ♦ exercise intensity
- ♦ duration of exercise
- ♦ frequency of exercise
- ♦ types of exercises

## Exercise Intensity

Most of us have had the experience of climbing stairs to the third story of an office or apartment building. As we get to the top, we stop to catch our breath. Our hearts are racing and we are breathing hard and fast. We have experienced an intense physical activity. If you were to check your pulse, it might be beating at 180 beats per minute (bpm).

The intensity of exercise is measured by the heart rate.

**Did You Know?**

The heart of a young child can easily get up to 220 bpm!

To find a person's maximal heart rate, the following formula can be used:

$$220 - \text{age} = \text{maximal heart rate}$$

**Example 1:**

A 20-year-old person

220 – 20 = 200 beats per minute

220 – 20 = 200 beats per minute

200 X 90% = 180 beats per minute

Research indicates that improvements in the aerobic system happen when a person is exercising at an intensity level **of 60 to 90 percent of his maximal heart rate**. In Example 1, the formula indicates that this person should exercise at an intensity level high enough so that the heart rate does not go below 120 beats per minute, but does not exceed 180 beats per minute. This is called the **target heart rate training zone (TZ).**

An unfit person should train at a lower intensity level (60%). A fit person can exercise at a higher intensity level (70 to 80%).

### TAKING YOUR PULSE

Our heart rates can be detected by our pulse. It is easiest to find your pulse on your neck. Place two fingers just under the jaw, about one inch in front of your ear. To find your **resting pulse rate**, sit in a chair and relax. Count the number of pulse beats for one minute straight. **This is your resting heart rate in beats per minute (bpm).**

To determine the intensity level of exercise, count the pulse rate during exercise. Stop exercising and immediately find the heart beat. (It should be easy when the heart is pounding.) Count the beats for 6 seconds; multiply by 10 to get beats per minute.

## Duration of Exercise

Improvement in aerobic capacity begins after 5 minutes of keeping the heart rate in the "target zone," and should continue for at least 10 minutes. A typical exercise plan has a goal of 60 minutes of exercise per week.

**To maintain a** healthy cardiovascular system, a child needs to elevate his heart rate for 10 to 20 minutes, three to six times a week, for a total of 60 minutes a week.

## Frequency of Exercise

Research indicates that to receive the maximal effects of aerobic exercise, it should be done at a minimum of once every 48 hours. Engaging in aerobic training between three to six times a week is recommended.

The examples of Johnny and Jane, below, illustrate the flexibility a person can have in establishing their own frequency.

**Johnny** exercises 15 minutes a day on Mon, Wed, Fri, Sat for 60 minutes a week.

**Jane** exercises 20 minutes a day on Mon, Wed, Fri for 60 minutes a week.

## TYPES OF EXERCISES THAT ARE AEROBIC

Activities like a 100-meter dash or weight lifting do not keep the heart rate elevated for 5 minutes, so these types of activities are not good aerobic exercises.

A good aerobic activity is one which elevates the heart rate and maintains the heart rate within the target training zone for at least 10 minutes.

Good examples of these activities are: soccer, swimming, bicycling, running, skipping rope, racquetball, cross-country skiing, and aerobic dance. It is important to choose activities that are enjoyable, and for which equipment or facilities are easily accesible.

◇◇◇◇◇◇◇◇◇◇◇◇◇◇◇◇◇◇◇◇◇◇◇◇◇◇◇◇◇◇◇◇

**The Favorite Aerobic** Activities of Children
Grades 1 to 4 in the USA
    Swimming
    Running
    Bicycling
    Soccer

◇◇◇◇◇◇◇◇◇◇◇◇◇◇◇◇◇◇◇◇◇◇◇◇◇◇◇◇◇◇◇◇

## Exercise Points

How much exercise is enough? As stated above, 60 minutes a week of aerobic exercise is a good start.

Children and adults who consistently exercise vigorously 60 minutes per week will probably attain a healthy fitness level. But how do you know if the *type* of exercise you are doing is adequate to attain physical fitness?

Rather than just keeping track of time spent exercising, exercise points should be used. The exercise points take into consideration the intensity of the activity *and* the duration of time doing the activity. In addition, the point system is a good tool for teaching older children (ages 9 and up) how the body responds to training. This information will also make their lifetime habit of exercise most effective.

Exercise points are computed at the conclusion of exercise, and recorded. Consistently exercising at a level of 300 points per week would put you in a superior fitness level, 200 points per week in an average level, and 100 points per week in a low fitness level.

Exercising above 300 points per week will increase aerobic capacity but will not necessarily improve general health and wellness. I recommend that the maximum point goal be 300 points per week—in other words, do not go above 300 points per week. (A serious athlete might have reasons to go over 300 points a week, but this is not necessary for the purposes of introducing your child to fitness).

## READING THE EXERCISE POINTS CHART

The exercise points chart I have included at the end of this chapter is a tool that allows you to participate in a variety of activities, and measure the amount of exercise you accomplish in each one.

For example:

You biked 2 miles in 9 minutes. In the exercise diary, you would record:

♦ the date
♦ type of activity (biking)
♦ distance (2 miles)
♦ duration (9 minutes)
♦ aerobic points obtained (10 points). (Use the biking chart at the end of this chapter to determine the number of points earned.)

Another day that week, you swim and earn 40 aerobic points. Also on another day, you jump rope and earn 60 points. At the end of each week you will total your points.

In this example, you would have 110 aerobic points for the week.

| Activity | Date | Distance | Duration | Points | Total |
|---|---|---|---|---|---|
| Bike | 3–1 | 2 mile | 9 min | 10 | 10 |
| Swim | 3–3 | 1600 yds | 60 min | 40 | 50 |
| Jump rope | 3–6 | | 20 min | 60 | 110 |

## SELECTING ACTIVITIES ON THE EXERCISE POINTS CHART

When selecting an activity from the exercise points chart, select those that are most enjoyable and for which you have access to the necessary equipment or facilities. To keep your child's interest high, allow him or her to choose which activities he or she wants.

Record the activity and points earned each day. Increase weekly totals by 10 points each week. This slow progression is attainable and should eliminate muscle soreness and injuries. Consistency is the key for improvement!

**Please note:** being disciplined and keeping an exercise journal is educational, but it need not be done all the time. For children younger than 9, recording time spent doing an activity is adequate. (If you have children between the ages of 4 to 8, go to the Lab: Aerobic Exercise Plan Ages 4 to 8, for an appropriate exercise schedule for this age group.)

## REWARDS

You can be creative in designing a reward system to use when your child reaches certain exercise points goals. For the child starting at a low fitness level, you may challenge her to increase the points she gets each week. If she continually improves her weekly point values for 10 consecutive weeks, she will be rewarded. For a child already starting at 300 points per week,

you can reward him for 10 consecutive weeks of maintaining this point level.

You may vary the reward and the weeks needed for rewards. The key is consistency and progress. I would encourage you to make a rule that your child cannot credit himself for more than 150 points in one day. This rule will help your child work toward more consistency in exercise.

### A Note on Consistency

Aches, pains, and injuries occur when the intensity or duration of an exercise is increased dramatically and sporadically. If a child misses 2 weeks of exercise, he will be unable to safely return to the same intensity or duration level of exercise that he had previously. Consistency is important!

At the end of this chapter you will find blank exercise Aerobic Plans and blank Exercise Point Charts for you to fill in with your children.

## GENERAL CAUTIONS AND TIPS
## Cold Weather

Exercising in cold weather is not generally harmful to a healthy person. The body produces heat when exercising and stays warm.

However, windchill and frostbite on exposed skin are a concern. Ears and fingers should be covered to protect from frostbite.

Keep in mind that, in the winter, the day is warmest between noon and three o'clock, so you may want to send children outside to exercise during this time.

Always, discretion and common sense should be used if windchill is below zero.

## Hot Weather

The body cools itself in hot weather by sweating: when sweat evaporates on the skin, it cools the body.

However, the combination of high temperature and high humidity lowers the body's ability to cool itself. Symptoms of heat-related illness can include weakness, headache, dizziness, and nausea. If you notice these symptoms, stop the activity and be sure your child rests in a cool place and drinks fluids.

Avoid the hottest part of the day by planning exercise for the morning or evening. You can also have the children play in the shade of a tree or house. Loose cotton and light-colored clothing will help the body stay cooler. Drinking plenty of water before and after exercise is also important (avoid very cold or sweetened drinks).

**As parents, we** need to actively encourage our children to drink extra fluids when they exercise, no matter what time of year. This is important because your child's own thirst level may not indicate the actual need for water.

## Shoes

Good shoes are important for active children. Poorly fitting shoes can cause blisters and do not provide adequate ankle support. In addition, shoes without a high, firm arch support or sole cushioning can cause shin splints or a heel bruise.

A guide to choosing appropriate shoes for various athletic purposes could take up a whole chapter just by itself! For the purposes of the activities in this book, however, I feel that a well-fit "cross trainer" is appropriate.

## Sore Muscles

Most soreness and injury can be eliminated by *slowly* increasing the intensity, duration, and frequency of physical activity. As stated earlier in this chapter, be sure to plan on consistent exercise, and always slowly increase the level of difficulty.

## HOW TO ENJOY EXERCISE AS A FAMILY

Here are some ideas that our family has tried to make aerobics a fun family activity. Once your children have been active with you, it will be easier to start them on their own more personalized program.

- The children join Mom when she does her aerobic exercises to a video tape.
- In the summer, we plan a brisk family walk after dinner. The children sometimes choose to ride in a stroller, Rollerblade, or ride a bike. We stop at two small parks on our walk, and the children play for 5 minutes on the equipment. We all look forward to the time together.

- Mom likes to jog outside in the early morning. She asks one of our sons to go with her to be her "bodyguard." The older sons jog with her, and the younger sons ride their bikes while she jogs. This makes them feel important and gives them one extra reason to exercise.

- Our children love it when Dad joins them in an activity. They love to have me play basketball, football, or soccer with them. Actually, any activity I join them in is fun for them (and me).

- We have planned special family exercise outings, or play games. We go biking, hiking along a river, or play capture the flag in our yard.

- We swim as a family once a week. (We swim with Grandma, whose apartment complex has an indoor pool). We spend 20 minutes giving lessons and swimming laps, and practicing all the strokes. The rest of the time we play games in the pool (Marco Polo, 500 Baseball, tag, splash the brother, etc.).

- I teach elementary exercise classes through our local community recreation department. I have taught soccer, kickball, volleyball, tennis, basketball, football, floor hockey, and bowling. Our community recreation department has had winter family gym nights, where parents and children play together with the balls and equipment. You could ask your recreation department to offer these types of classes or open gym time. A church with a gym may be another resource.

- Invite friends over with the intent to play an aerobic game (tag, capture the flag).

- Get a jump rope for each family member and have a jump rope competition.

- See the activities marked as aerobic in Chapter 4: Modified Games, for more ideas.

## HOW TO START AND MAINTAIN AN AEROBIC EXERCISE PLAN

You have learned the basic principles of aerobic exercise and introduced your child to family aerobic activity through some of the suggestions above. Now you can develop a specific plan tailored to your child's interests.

Be aware that many people drop out of an exercise program after the first month. Why? They lose interest. Avoid this common pitfall by choosing several enjoyable activities. Once you and your child get past the first month, exercise will begin to become a habit, and this can bring great personal satisfaction.

### Here are some tips to get you started—and keep you going:

1. Use a combination of activities. I encourage you to do at least two different activities each week. Doing the same activity day after day can get boring.

2. Plan! If you do not have a plan it is easier to skip your exercises. Put exercise in your daily class schedule. The schedule and types of activities may vary with the seasons, but always have a time and day planned.

3. Have the right equipment. Get good shoes. Have balls or mitts in a special place (trunk, closet) where they are always returned after play. This will save time and reduce frustration.

**4.** Keep a written record of activity, so you will be able to observe the child's progress and compare previous months and years. After exercising has become a habit, daily record keeping may not be needed.

**5.** Make exercising a positive experience. Be creative in ways to make it fun, and reward good work.

## LAB: TARGET HEART RATE

Name: _____  Age: _____  Date: _____

Two basic factors enter into computing your estimated safe exercise zone; these are age and lifestyle. Use the formula below to compute your target heart rate for your aerobic activities.

**1.** Compute your estimated maximal heart rate (MHR). Formula = 220 – age = MHR
220 – (your age) _____ = (MHR) _____ Beats per minute (bpm)

**2.** Compute your target heart rate. MHR x intensity percentage = Target Heart Rate (THR)

Individuals who have not been physically active should start exercising at the 60% intensity level and slowly increase the intensity level. Individuals who are already fit should start at the 70% intensity level and increase slowly toward the 90% intensity level. Choose the level that is appropriate for you (60%, 70%, 80%, 90%) and place it in the formula below.

Your MHR _____ X _____% = _____ target heart rate in beats per minute.

**3.** My heart rate during exercise should stay around _____ beats per minute.

◇◇◇◇◇◇◇◇◇◇◇◇◇◇◇◇◇◇◇◇◇◇◇◇◇◇◇◇◇◇◇◇◇◇◇◇◇◇◇◇◇◇◇◇◇◇◇◇◇◇◇◇◇◇◇◇◇◇◇◇◇◇◇◇◇◇◇◇◇◇◇◇◇◇◇◇◇◇

**My Target Heart** Rate Range is _____ beats per minute in six seconds, the count should be _____ beats per minute

◇◇◇◇◇◇◇◇◇◇◇◇◇◇◇◇◇◇◇◇◇◇◇◇◇◇◇◇◇◇◇◇◇◇◇◇◇◇◇◇◇◇◇◇◇◇◇◇◇◇◇◇◇◇◇◇◇◇◇◇◇◇◇◇◇◇◇◇◇◇◇◇◇◇◇◇◇◇

# LAB: AEROBIC EXERCISE PLAN

## AGES 4–8

Name: _____ Age: _____ Date: _____

## Purpose

To provide the parent with an objective measurement of his child's exercise level.

Is your 4 to 8 year old getting enough exercise? Young children love to run and play. They normally will get enough exercise if we provide them the opportunity. Record on the chart below the approximate number of minutes of vigorous physical activity your child obtains in one week.

|  | Monday | Tuesday | Wednesday | Thursday | Friday | Saturday | Sunday |
|---|---|---|---|---|---|---|---|
| Type of activity |  |  |  |  |  |  |  |
| Minutes of activity |  |  |  |  |  |  |  |

1. My child is currently getting _____ minutes of vigorous exercise each week.
2. My child will increase to 60 minutes of vigorous exercise each week.
3. My child plans to do the following family aerobic activities this month (pick an activity and a date) _____ , _____ , _____ , _____ .
4. Have the child list the activities he would like to do consistently this month. _____ , _____ , _____ , _____ .
5. I plan to enable my child to do these activities during the following days of the week. (circle)

   **Mon    Tues    Wed    Thurs    Fri    Sat    Sun**
6. My child's target heart rate is _____ . (optional)
7. On the 1-Mile Run/Walk Test, my child traveled 1 mile in _____ minutes.

   (Optional) You may give your child the 1-Mile Run/Walk Test as described in the "Tests" chapter. The time listed on the 1- Mile Run/Walk charts is the time your child must meet or exceed to be at a healthy fitness level.
8. My child's time was better than the recommended minimal fitness score. (circle one) Yes No

# LAB: AEROBIC EXERCISE PLAN

## AGE 9 and UP

Name: _____ Age: _____ Date: _____

## Purpose

To provide the parent with an objective measurement of his child's exercise level.

This lab is to be done by the child with guidance from the parent.

Are you getting enough exercise? By this age, habits of life have begun to set in. Record on the chart below the approximate number of minutes of vigorous physical activity you obtain in one week.

| | Monday | Tuesday | Wednesday | Thursday | Friday | Saturday | Sunday |
|---|---|---|---|---|---|---|---|
| Type of activity | | | | | | | |
| Minutes of activity | | | | | | | |

1. I am currently getting _____ minutes of vigorous exercise each week.
2. Do the 1-Mile Run/Walk test as described in the "Tests" chapter.
3. My time on the 1-Mile Run/Walk test was better than the recommended minimal fitness score for my age.        (circle one)     Yes     No
4. If your time was faster than the time listed for your age, then you are at a healthy fitness level. As your times improve, you will move to a higher fitness level.
5. I plan to do the following aerobic activities by myself and with others this month.

   _____ , _____ , _____ , _____ .

6. I plan to do these activities during the following days of the week. (circle)
   **Mon     Tues     Wed     Thurs     Fri     Sat     Sun**
7. Read the section in this chapter labeled "Reading The Exercise Charts." Begin recording your exercise points in the exercise journal. (The exercise charts and journal are located at the end of this chapter.)
8. In my first week of recording exercise points, I scored _____ points.
9. I plan to increase 10 exercise points per week.
10. My target heart rate from the previous lab is _____ .
12. I will show one person _____ my exercise log periodically to be accountable to them.

# EXERCISE POINTS CHARTS

The purpose of the exercise charts is to obtain a weekly total of points, which represent the quantity of aerobic activity. The points allow you to measure the amount of exercise you have obtained even though you participate in a variety of activities at a variety of intensity levels. After you have done aerobic activity, compute the aerobic points you obtained and record the points on your Exercise Points Journal (end of this chapter.) The chart below lists aerobic activities and the number of points you receive for each 10 minutes of doing the activity.

| Activity | Points |
|---|---|
| Aerobic Dance Beginner Level | 20 |
| Aerobic Dance Intermediate Level | 30 |
| Basketball* | 15 |
| Cross-Country Skiing | 30 |
| Cycling-Stationary Moderate speed 60 Rpm/18 Mph | 20 |
| Handball | 15 |
| Hockey | 15 |
| Ice Skating** | 8 |
| Lacrosse | 15 |
| Mini-trampoline | 6 |
| Racquetball | 15 |
| Rollerblading | 8 |
| Roller Skating | 8 |
| Rope Jumping 70–90 steps / min | 30 |
| Rope Jumping 90–110 steps/min*** | 40 |
| Rowing Machine | 20 |
| Running-Stationary 60–70 steps/min† | 20 |
| Running-Stationary 80–90 steps/min† | 40 |
| Soccer | 15 |
| Squash | 15 |
| Stair-climbing | 15 |
| Tennis/Badminton Singles | 6 |
| Tennis/Badminton Doubles | 3 |
| Volleyball | 5 |
| Water/Downhill Skiing | 6 |

| * | Continuous exercise. Do not count breaks or time-outs. |
| --- | --- |
| ** | For competitive speed skating triple the point value. |
| *** | Skip with both feet together or step over the rope, alternating feet. |
| † | Count only the left foot. Raise the feet approximately 8 inches off the floor. |

## Exercise Point Charts for activities with a known distance

| Cycling 2 miles* | 11 min | 10 |
| | 7 min | 20 |
| | under 6 min | 30 |
| | | |
| Golf** | 9 holes | 15 |
| | 18 holes | 30 |
| | | |
| Running/Walking 1 mile | 20 min | 10 |
| | 14 min | 20 |
| | 11 min | 30 |
| | 9 min | 40 |
| | 7 | 50 |
| | below | 60 |
| Swimming 400 yards (crawl stroke, back stroke, butterfly) | 14 min | 10 |
| | 12 min | 15 |
| | 8 min | 35 |

\*   If using more than a 3-speed or 10-speed bike deduct 20%.

\*\*  No motorized carts.

**note:** The point charts for roller blading are similar to walking. You need to rollerblade twice as fast as you jog in order to get the same amount of exercise. Most people Rollerblade at a speed of twice as fast as walking. For games listed in the "Games" chapter, award yourself 10 points for each 10 minutes of activity.

## EXAMPLE

| Activity | Date | Distance | Time | Pts | Cum Pts |
|----------|------|----------|------|-----|---------|
| Bike | 3–1 | 2 mile | 9 min | 10 | 10 |
| Swim | 3–3 | 1600 yds | 60 min | 40 | 50 |
| Jump rope | 3–6 | | 20 min | 60 | 110 |

# EXERCISE POINTS JOURNAL

Name: _____  Age: _____  For the month of: _____

| Date | Exercise | Distance (miles or yards) | Time (minutes) | Points | Weekly Point Totals |
|------|----------|---------------------------|----------------|--------|---------------------|
| 1 | | | | | |
| 2 | | | | | |
| 3 | | | | | |
| 4 | | | | | |
| 5 | | | | | |
| 6 | | | | | |
| 7 | | | | | |
| 8 | | | | | |
| 9 | | | | | |
| 10 | | | | | |
| 11 | | | | | |
| 12 | | | | | |
| 13 | | | | | |
| 14 | | | | | |
| 15 | | | | | |
| 16 | | | | | |
| 17 | | | | | |
| 18 | | | | | |
| 19 | | | | | |
| 20 | | | | | |
| 21 | | | | | |
| 22 | | | | | |
| 23 | | | | | |
| 24 | | | | | |
| 25 | | | | | |
| 26 | | | | | |
| 27 | | | | | |
| 28 | | | | | |
| 29 | | | | | |
| 30 | | | | | |
| 31 | | | | | |

Photocopy this page for your exercise journal. Record the activity, time you did the activity, and exercise points from the aerobic exercise charts. See previous page for an example. Total your points weekly. The goal is to consistently increase the weekly total.

# TEST QUESTIONS

Give this test to your child and score it. Answers are at the bottom of the page.

John Doe's dad felt that he needed to improve his cardiovascular fitness. His father jogged with him daily.

**1.** How could John know if he was jogging vigorously enough to improve his fitness?
   a. if he started sweating
   b. if his heart rate increased to 160 beats per minute
   c. if he started breathing hard
   d. if his legs started to get tired

**2.** Which would be a good test for John to see how fit his cardiovascular system was?
   a. sit-up test
   b. 100-meter run
   c. pull-up test
   d. 1-mile run

**3.** What kind of exercise did John do?
   a. aerobic exercise
   b. isometric exercise
   c. anaerobic exercise
   d. stretching exercise

**4.** How often should John exercise aerobically?
   a. once a week
   b. three times a month
   c. three times a week
   d. four times a month

**5.** When John plans his aerobic fitness program, the first thing he should do is what?
   a. compute his target heart rate training zone
   b. list his attitudes about exercise
   c. list the facilities available
   d. list the activities he likes to do

**6.** Sedentary people usually have resting heart rates that are:
   a. higher than physically active people
   b. lower than physically active people
   c. same as physically active people

**7.** The average resting heart rate for a young adult is about:
   a. 50 beats per minute
   b. 70 beats per minute
   c. 100 beats per minute

**8.** A student will meet the aerobically healthy standard with _____ minutes of aerobic activity per week.
   a. 30
   b. 60
   c. 90
   d. 120

**Answers:** 1a, 2d, 3a, 4c, 5a, 6a, 7b, 8b

## Key Terms

**Aerobic Exercise**—Continuous exercise that can be maintained beyond 5 minutes. The body is able to keep up with the demand for oxygen. Examples: jogging, soccer, swimming. The body utilizing oxygen to supply the body with energy.

**Anaerobic Exercise**—All-out exercise lasting 20–40 seconds. The muscles use oxygen faster than the body can supply it. Example; weight lifting, sprints, volleyball. The body creates energy by a process that does not use oxygen.

**Body composition**—The percentage of body fat.

**Calisthenics**—Various exercises utilizing both aerobic and anaerobic fitness exercises.

**Cardiovascular efficiency**—The ability of the heart to deliver oxygen to all of the vital organs of the body.

**Cooling down**—Continuation of exercise at a low intensity level following strenuous exercise to allow the body to adjust to normal resting levels.

**Flexibility**—The extent and range of motion around a joint.

**Health-related fitness**—Those aspects of our physical and psychological makeup that afford us some protection against coronary heart diseases, muscle and joint ailments, and various other diseases.

**Static stretching**—A stretching method that consists of stretching the muscles slowly, and holding the stretch for 5–60 seconds.

**Warm-up**—Exercises performed immediately before physical activity to prepare the heart, lungs, and muscles to adequately meet the demands of rigorous exercise.

# Modified Fitness Games with Minimal Equipment

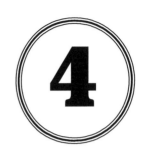

LISTED BELOW ARE some fitness games we have enjoyed with our own children. They can all be played at home, with a minimal amount of equipment, and each game encourages physical fitness. Some are traditional games and others, we created. They can all be played as a family or with a small group of children (please note an adult should always supervise).

The games are divided into three categories: indoor games, outdoor games, and snow games.

These games have been specifically selected for their value in teaching certain skills. The following three charts summarize which skills are utilized in each game. These charts can be used in conjunction with the lessons in chapter 6 to help you determine which games are appropriate to build the desired skill set.

**Tip:** Many of these games can be played during social events. My wife uses games in this chapter for birthday parties and family reunions.

◇◇◇◇◇◇◇◇◇◇◇◇◇◇◇◇◇◇◇◇◇◇◇◇◇◇◇◇◇◇

**The next time** your child says, "I'm bored,"
have him try one of these games.

◇◇◇◇◇◇◇◇◇◇◇◇◇◇◇◇◇◇◇◇◇◇◇◇◇◇◇◇◇◇

## INDOOR/OUTDOOR GAMES

1. **Simon Says (movement)**—One person is chosen to be "Simon" and the other players stand in a straight line. Simon then calls out a command for the children to follow. Simon should only be obeyed if he prefaces his statement with "Simon says." For example, if Simon says "touch your nose" without first saying, "Simon says," then no one should touch their nose. Whoever does touch their nose is out. The last child standing becomes the new Simon. Suggested "commands" to encourage physical activity include jumping jacks, kangaroo jumps, etc.
   - Equipment: none
   - Two or more players

2. **Follow The Leader (aerobic)**—This game can be played indoors or outdoors. Players follow the leader and imitate whatever he or she does. Activities to encourage physical activity include sprinting, climbing trees, hopping . . . the only limit is your imagination!
   - Equipment: none
   - Two or more players

3. **Forty Ways to Get There (movement)**—This game can be played easily in any room of the home, or in a set area outdoors. Each player takes turns moving from one end of the room to the other. Once a type of movement has been used by one player (walking, hopping, skipping, crawling, etc.) that movement cannot be used again. Game continues until a player cannot think of a new way to move.
   - Equipment: none
   - Two or more players

4. **Four Square (striking)**—Locate an area of pavement (in a basement, driveway, or local park) and use chalk or tape to mark a square approximately 16 feet wide. Divide square into four equal four-by-four foot squares. Label the squares A, B, C, and D.

| A | D |
|---|---|
| B | C |

   - Equipment: tape or chalk; 8-inch playground rubber ball
   - Two or more players

   **How to Play:**
   1. One player stands in each square.
   2. The person standing in the A square always starts the game. Bounce the ball, then hit once with the hand (or hands) in the direction of another square. The goal is to get the ball to bounce in another square.
   3. The player standing in the square where the ball ends up must hit it after *only one* bounce, into any of the other three squares.
   4. The game proceeds until one player

fails to hit the ball, or fails to hit the ball into another player's square.

5. After each round, the player who fails to return the ball properly goes to the D square. Other players move closer to the A position.

The goal of the game is to stay in the A square as long as possible.

**Rules:**

6. The ball must be hit with an upward motion of the hands.

7. No spiking or hitting the ball with a fist is allowed.

8. Ball cannot be held.

9. Lines are out of bounds.

10. A always starts the game.

11. If the player is standing in his square and is struck with the ball, he goes to the D square.

12. If the player is standing outside his square and is struck with the ball, the player who passed the ball goes to the D square.

**Variation:** Instead of the bounce-and-hit, have the player catch the ball after it bounces in their square. This is good for younger children first learning the game.

**5. Hopscotch (coordination)**—Mark squares on a floor or driveway with chalk or tape.

- Equipment: tape or chalk; flat stone or other object that can be tossed onto pavement
- Two or more players.

**How to Play:**

The player tosses the stone onto a square, beginning with 1. The player hops on one foot to the square where the stone landed. in each single square, and one foot in each square in adjacent squares (left foot in 4 and right foot in 5). When the player gets to squares 7 and 8, he must jump up and turn around in the air and land with feet in the squares 7 and 8. The player hops back to the start. The players must modify their hopping so they do not land in the square with the stone in it. On the return trip, the player must stop in the square before the puck, bend over and pick up the puck, then continue hopping back to the starting point.

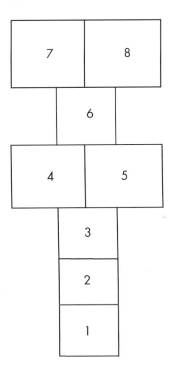

**6. Balloon Volleyball (hand/eye coordination)**—Set up two chairs across from each other and stretch a string between the two chairs. Have the players bat a beach ball or balloon over the string. Count how many times the ball can be passed back and forth in the air before hitting the floor.

HOME SCHOOL FAMILY FITNESS

- Equipment: string, chairs, balloon or beach ball
- Two or more players

**Variation**

Use a ruler or paddle to strike the balloon back and forth over the string. This will help improve striking skills used in sports like baseball and tennis.

7. **Indoor Mini-basketball (shooting)**—Place a trash can or other container along the wall. Players take turns shooting beanbags or rolled up socks into the trash can from a free-throw line. Count who makes the most baskets.
   - Equipment: trash can or other container, beanbags or rolled-up socks
   - One or more players

8. **Pin Guard (throwing)**—Draw, or mark with tape, a circle 6 to 10 feet in diameter. A player stands in the middle. A milk carton is placed in the middle of the circle. One or more players stand outside the circle. They try to knock the milk carton down using a Nerf ball or rolled up sock. They may toss the ball around or across the circle to each other to get a better shot at the milk carton. The player in the middle of the circle tries to guard the milk carton and keep it from being knocked down. Whoever succeeds in knocking down the milk carton becomes the new guard. If the guard knocks the milk carton over himself, he chooses another player to be the new guard.
   - Equipment: milk carton, Nerf ball or rolled up sock
   - Two or more players

9. **Dodgeball (throwing, dodging)**—Choose an area to play where balls can be thrown (garage, basement, local park). Players stand in front of a wall with one player facing them. The players in front of the wall try to dodge balls thrown at them by one player. The thrower gets one point for each time he hits a player. Rotate throwers every 2 minutes.
   - Caution: Hits on the head do not count, and should be discouraged to avoid injury.
   - Equipment: Nerf balls
   - Two or more players.

   **Variation:** In this variation, the parent throws the balls. Mark two squares on the ground at opposite ends of the wall. These squares are "safe zones" where the player cannot be hit. The children run from box to box, dodging the balls as they are thrown. The child earns one point for each time he makes it to a box without getting hit. The thrower earns one point for each time he hits the runner. This variation makes the game a better aerobic activity.

10. **Keep Away (throwing, catching)**—Players should form two teams. One team passes the ball back and forth, while the other team tries to intercept it. Two balls can be used for a more fast-paced game.
    - Equipment: soft ball or object, or rolled up sock
    - Three or more players

11. **Blanket Toss (hand/eye coordination)**—Children and parents hold the edge of a blanket or sheet. In the middle, put a beach ball, table tennis ball, or foam ball. Pull up and down on the sheet, tossing the ball into the air and catching it again in the sheet. See how many times you can

toss the ball up without letting it hit the ground.

- Equipment: Blanket or sheet, beach ball, table tennis ball, foam ball, or rolled up sock
- Three or more players

12. **Flashlight Tag (movement, muscle endurance)**—A large room is needed for this game. Arrange chairs, sofas, and sofa cushions in a scattered formation around the room. You can also drape blankets over folding chairs. The person with the flashlight sits in a chair at one end of the room. A pillow is placed on the floor 3 feet in front of the person with the flashlight. The other players stand at the opposite end of the room. The lights are turned off. The other players try to hide behind the obstacles and advance forward toward the pillow, while the person with the flashlight tries to catch their faces in the beam of light. A person is eliminated if they are caught in the flashlight and his or her name is called out. The first player to get to the pillow without being caught becomes the new flashlight holder.

    **Hint:** Turn on some music to help muffle the sounds of the players moving around; this will make it harder for the person with the flashlight to spot them.

    - Equipment: Large room with furniture; pillow; flashlight
    - Three or more players

13. **Tiger Tails (aerobic)**—Tuck a tube sock or handkerchief in the waistband of each player so the tube sock or handkerchief hangs out like a "tail." The object is to snatch someone else's tails while protecting your own.

    - Equipment: tube sock or handkerchief
    - Two or more players

    **With two players:** stop the action when one tail is snatched, and award one point to the snatcher.

    **With three or more players:** stop the action after all tails have been snatched and award points for the number of tails each player has taken. (If a player loses his tail, he may continue to play.)

14. **Fox and Rabbit (catching, throwing)**—Four or more players sit in a circle. One beanbag, called the "rabbit" is passed around the circle. A second beanbag, called "fox," is passed around the circle next. When the fox catches the rabbit, the game ends.

    - Equipment: beanbags
    - Four or more players

15. **Floor Tennis (striking)**—With chalk or tape, mark lines approximately the size of a ping-pong table on the ground or floor. Place a string between two chairs approximately 12 inches high. Hang newspaper over the string to make the net. Follow ping-pong tennis rules.

    - Equipment: Ping-pong paddles and ping-pong (or paper cup and folded up newspapers or magazines), chairs, string, newspaper
    - Two to four players

16. **Badminiature (striking)**—With chalk or tape, make court boundaries using two boxes approximately 5 feet square. Stretch a string between two chairs 2 to 3 feet high. Follow badminton rules. If you do not have badminton rackets and a

shuttlecock, a paper cup can be used as a shuttlecock and folded magazines or cardboard can be used as paddles.

- Equipment: Ping-pong paddles and ping-pong (or, paper cup and folded up newspapers or magazines), chairs, string, newspaper
- Two to four players

17. **Beanbag Toss (throwing)**—Assign the children after a meal to make 25 baskets by tossing the beanbag into an empty trash can. The first person to make 25 baskets gets to choose their after-meal dessert. One or more players.

18. **Sardines**—This game requires an area where several players can hide in the dark, but be sure an adult checks the area where play will occur to confirm it is safe, first. The game begins when one person hides and the others quietly look for him or her. When a seeker finds the "sardine," the seeker quietly hides with the sardine. More and more players will be hidden together. The last person to find the sardine is the new sardine.

- Three or more players

19. **Obstacle Course (coordination/endurance)**—A course can be set up indoors or outdoors. Be creative when you set up the course. Examples: a 2x4 board can be set up for children to walk across like a balance beam, or they can jump high over tape between two chairs. Some activities to complete can include: forward rolls; backward rolls; and toss the ball up, spin once, and catch the ball. Time how fast they can race through the course. Have the children start at different stations of the course and try to catch up and tag a person ahead of them.

- Equipment: various furniture and objects to set up an obstacle course
- One or more players

20. **Can Race (coordination)**—All players line up on a starting line. Each player should already be balancing on one tin can, and holding an extra tin can. At the starting signal, each player places the extra can in front of her and steps onto it. Then, she reaches behind her to retrieve the other can, and moves forward step by step. In this way, without touching the ground, each player slowly advances until they cross the finish line. If a player falls or any part of his body touches the ground, he or she must start over at the starting line.

**Variation**

Use a square piece of cardboard instead of cans.

- Equipment: tin cans or cardboard
- Two or more players

21. **Wild Ball (coordination/striking)**—Players begin on their hands and knees in a bedroom or family room. One soft foam ball is placed in the middle of the room. At the "go" command, players move as fast as they can towards the ball, moving on their hands and knees. The ball can only be struck with the hand, and cannot be held or caught. A player is eliminated if the ball touches any other part of the body. When a player is eliminated, play stops and the game begins again with one less person, until only one person is left.

**Hint:** A good way to eliminate someone is to bounce the ball off the wall to hit him or her.

**Variation**—Two teams. Divide the room in half with a towel. Same rules as above, except if the ball stops rolling on your half, a player is eliminated on your side.

**Variation**—Divide the room in half. One person (superman) plays against all other players. Superman stays on his half of the room and the other players stay on their half. The player who eliminates "superman" becomes superman next.

**Variation**—with ages 13 and up, play standing up instead of on the knees (it is more comfortable).

- Equipment: soft foam ball
- Two or more players

22. **Fool Ball (catching)**—Players form a circle with one player in the middle. The player in the middle holds a Nerf ball. The players in the circle have their hands behind their backs. The person in the middle begins throwing the ball clockwise in order of the people in the circle. The player in the middle may fake throwing. Any player who takes his hands out from behind his back to catch the ball when the ball is not being thrown to him, is eliminated.
    - Equipment: ball
    - Three or more players

23. **Musical Balloons (catching)**—Similar to musical chairs. The players stand in a circle, with everyone holding a balloon except for one person. When the music starts playing, the balloons are passed in a clockwise direction around the circle. When the music stops, the person without a balloon is out. If a balloon pops, the person holding it is out.
    - Equipment: balloon

- Three or more players

24. **Car**—A tag game using remote control cars. Players run in a bedroom or family room avoiding being touched by the car. When they are touched by the car they are eliminated or are given a point. The winner is the last one standing or the person with the least points. Rotate who operates the car.
    - Equipment: One or two remote control cars (preferably the kind that keeps going when it flips over) depending upon the number of people.

25. **Hack Four Square**—This game is played like four square, with a hackysack instead of a rubber ball. The hackysack must be kept in the air while being passed from square to square. If the receiver fails to hit the hackysack and it lands in his square, or lands out of bounds after he touches it, he is out. The hackysack must always be hit in upward direction at a distance of at least 6 inches off the ground.
    - Equipment: hackysack
    - Two or more players

## OUTDOOR GAMES

1. **Anti-I-Over (throwing, catching)**—Form two teams. Play with one tennis ball. The teams stand on opposite sides of the garage or house. Team A with the ball shouts "Anti-I-Over" and throws the ball over the garage. If the ball does not make it over the roof, Team A shouts "Pig's tails." If Team B catches the ball without bouncing, then Team B runs around the building and tries to tag the opponents

before they can run to the opposite side of the building. Each tagged player counts as one point. If Team B does not catch the ball before it bounces on the ground, they cannot tag opponents. They must then call out "Anti-I-Over" and throw the ball back over the building. An alternative tagging method is to hit the opponents with the ball (nerf or playground ball).

- Equipment: tennis ball
- Two or more players

2. **500 Baseball (ages 8 and up) (throwing, catching)**—A player is appointed as thrower. The thrower throws the ball into the air to a group of players downfield. If a player successfully catches the ball, he is awarded points in the following way:

- 100 points for a fly
- 50 points for one bounce
- 25 points for two bounces
- 10 points for a rolling ball.

If a player touches a ball but does not successfully catch it, he is awarded negative points. For example, a player who drops a fly ball is awarded a negative 100 points, and a player behind him who catches the ball on one bounce is awarded 50 points. The first player to score 500 is the new thrower.

**Variations:** for different grades:
Grades 1–4: kick a rubber utility ball
Grades 4 and up: throw a football instead of a baseball.

The scoring is the same for both variations.

- Equipment: baseball, baseball gloves (or equipment for variations listed above)
- Two or more players

3. **Home Run Baseball (aerobic, batting)**—Set the bases further apart than in standard baseball (this will bring more running into the game). The ball is pitched to a batter. When the ball is hit, the outfielder must get the ball and tag the runner or home plate before the batter runs around all the bases.

**Hint:** A group of children with varied ages can also play by setting up shorter bases for the younger kids and longer bases for the older ones.

**Variation:** All players must run backwards when fielding and running around bases.

- Equipment: baseball, baseball gloves, bat, and bases
- Two or more players

4. **Kickball (kicking, throwing, introduction to baseball)**—Kickball is a great way to introduce baseball rules to first graders. If you have only two or three players, you can use the same rules as Home Run Baseball. If you have eight or more, you can play regular kickball.

Grades K-6: Kickball rules are basically the same as baseball, except that the ball is pitched by rolling it across the plate (similar to bowling), and the ball is kicked rather than hit with a bat.

**Variation:** Mat Kickball: for eight or more players. You may have any number of people on a base. Base runners must round the bases twice before they can score. Example, before a runner can score he must go to 1st, 2nd, 3rd, 1st, 2nd, 3rd and then home. This keeps more people active during the game and avoids having bored children sitting on the bench.

**Variation:** Backward kickball: fielders must run backwards to field the ball and the batter must run backwards around the bases.

- Equipment: kickball
- Two or more players

5. **Speedy Soccer (aerobic, kicking, soccer skills)**—Divide into two teams. Set up goals at each end of the playing field using milk cartons or plastic pails. Play regular soccer but with no goal keeper. Play with a foam ball to reduce injuries. To increase activity, use two balls. Increase the challenge by using a tennis ball or wiffle ball.

- Equipment: milk cartons or plastic pails; waffle ball, foam ball, or tennis ball
- Two or more players

6. **Newcomb Volleyball (introduction to volleyball, catching, throwing)**—Stretch a rope between two chairs or trees. Use a beach ball or Nerf ball. Mark boundaries for a court. Play volleyball, but instead of spiking the ball, have the players catch and throw the ball over the rope. Count how many times you can volley the ball across the rope before it touches the ground.

Grades K-4: Younger children can let the ball bounce once before they catch it and throw the ball back over the net.

**Hint:** Different ages can play together if the younger children are allowed to catch and throw the ball while the older ones must use regular volleyball hits. (Usually children are in fifth grade before they have the skills to successfully play regular volleyball.)

- Equipment: chairs, rope, beach ball or soft foam ball
- Four or more players

7. **Football Punt and Catch (kicking, catching)**—Grades 3–6: Mark three zones on a field, each approximately 20 feet square. The middle zone is the neutral zone. Divide into two teams. Team A punts the ball. If the ball lands or is caught in Team B's zone, Team A gets a point. If Team B catches the ball, Team B also gets a point. Team B then punts the ball back to Team A.

- Equipment: football
- Two or more players

```
┌─────────────┐
│   Team A    │
│    Zone     │
├─────────────┤
│   Neutral   │
│    Zone     │
├─────────────┤
│   Team B    │
│    Zone     │
└─────────────┘
```

8. **Frisbee Football (aerobic)**—Divide into two teams. Establish two goal lines. The goal is to get the Frisbee across the opponent's goal line by throwing the frisbee

to a teammate. The person throwing the Frisbee must remain stationary. If the Frisbee touches the ground, the other team takes possession of it. The Frisbee may be intercepted. A ball can be substituted for a Frisbee for younger players.

- Equipment: Frisbee
- Four or more players

9. **Kids' Handball (striking, hand/eye coordination, aerobic)**—This is handball (with modified rules) using an 8-inch rubber playground ball to slow the play down. Mark a handball court on the driveway in front of the garage door. The approximate dimensions are 8' wide, 10' deep, and a service line 5' from the garage. Player A serves the ball by letting it bounce once and hitting it with his hand. The ball must hit the wall and bounce in-bounds behind the service line. Player B must hit the ball after it bounces once and return the ball so it strikes the garage and bounces in-bounds anywhere in the court. After the service volley, the ball may bounce anywhere in the court, in front of or behind the service line. The opponent wins the serve if a player fails to return a ball before it bounces twice or he hits a ball out of bounds. A player can score points only when he is serving. If a player wins the serve when he is not serving, he gets the right to serve.

**Variation:** Three people play at once.

Note: Grades 3 to adult love this game! (Watch the children beat the adults.)

- Equipment: 8-inch rubber playground ball
- Two or more players

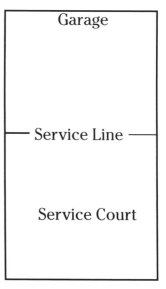

10. **Lightning Basketball (shooting, aerobic)**—Player A shoots a free throw and keeps shooting until he makes a basket. After the ball has left player A's hands, player B may shoot at the basket. If player B gets his ball in the basket before player A, player A is eliminated. When player A makes a basket, he passes the ball to player C, who is standing on the free throw line. Player C tries to make a basket before player B makes a basket. Repeat until only one player remains.

- Equipment: basketball
- Two or more players

11. **Deck Tennis (catching, throwing, aerobic)**—This is a modified form of tennis. Draw a court outline on the grass or driveway. (When playing with a group of children of different ages, the court dimensions may be smaller for younger players.) Deck rings are circular rings approximately 7 inches in diameter and can be purchased or made from rope or plastic tubing. The server must stand behind the

base line and on the right half of the court. He must throw the ring underhanded so that the ring travels upward in an arch to the other player, who is standing on the right side of the court. (The server must alternate courts on each serve.)

The receiver must catch the ring with one hand and, within three seconds, immediately return the ring to any part of the opponent's court. The server scores a point if the receiver fails to return the ring or commits a foul. Fouls are: catching a ring with two tennishands, changing the ring to the other hand before tossing it, holding the ring too long before returning it (that is, longer than three seconds,) stepping over the net or rope, the ring does not fly in an arc, or throwing the ring out of bounds. If the server misses the return, there is a change in servers but no points awarded. First player to get 11 points wins.

| Left Court | Right Court |
|---|---|
| Right Court | Left Court |

25 ft. (vertical, left side)

25 ft.      25 ft.

- Equipment: deck rings
- Two or four players

12. **Tug Of War (muscle strength/endurance)—** This game requires a sturdy rope 10 to 20 feet long. Divide into two teams. Both teams grab the rope at opposite ends and try to pull the opponents across a line. For excitement, make the line a soaker hose.
   - Equipment: sturdy 10 to 20 foot long rope
   - Two or more players

13. **Cops and Robbers (aerobic)—**Divide into two teams. Each person has a water gun or water balloons. If a player is shot, he must go to jail until a free partner tags him or the water on his clothes evaporates. The team that puts all their opponents in jail wins.
   - Equipment: water gun or water balloons
   - Four or more players

14. **Capture the Flag (aerobic)—**This is an all-time favorite! Divide into two teams. Divide the play area into two areas. Each team will hide a flag (red bandana) in their half of the playing field. (This obviously does not work well on an open field.) The object of the game is to find the opponent's flag and bring it back to your side of the playing field. If a player is tagged by an opponent while on the opponent's half of the playing field, he goes to jail. A player gets out of jail by being tagged by one of his teammates who is free. A prisoner who has been set free is given a "free trip home" to his half of the playing field. A variation is to get out of jail by counting to 500.
   - Equipment: red bandanas
   - Four or more players

15. **Hide and Seek (aerobic)—**One child is "it" and counts to 50 while the others hide. "It" looks for the "hiders". "Hiders" try to sneak back to a designated home base before "it" can tag them. The first child to

get to home base without being tagged is the next "it."

- Equipment: none
- Two or more players

16. **Freeze Tag (aerobic, dodging)**—Another all-time favorite! One or more players are selected as "it." "It" freezes people by tagging them or hitting them with foam balls. When a player is tagged, he must stand frozen and not move. A frozen player is unfrozen when someone crawls between his legs. The last one frozen is the new "it," or a new "it" can be chosen when the old one becomes exhausted. One way to give the players more activity is to let them unfreeze if they do calisthenics, such as 30 jumping jacks. Let the child's imagination modify the game.

- Equipment: none
- Four or more players

17. **Blob (aerobic)**—A person is appointed to be "it." When "it" tags another person, they join hands and try to tag another person. When they tag a third person, the three hold hands. When a fourth person is tagged, the blob splits in half and becomes two blobs. Any member of the blob may tag. As more people are tagged, more blobs are created. The last person to be tagged is the new "it" for the next game.

- Equipment: none
- Six or more players

18. **Marco Polo**—This game is played in a swimming pool. One person is appointed "it." "It" tries to tag other people while keeping his eyes closed. When "it" shouts "Marco" the other people must respond

and say "Polo." When a person is tagged, he becomes the new "it."

- Equipment: none
- Three or more players

19. **Snake Catch (aerobic, hand/eye coordination)**—One player is chosen to be the "snake holder" and is given a jump rope. The snake holder runs around the playing area dragging the free end of the rope on the ground. Other players try to catch the free end of the rope with their hands (the rope may not be stepped on.) The player who catches the rope becomes the new snake holder.

- Equipment: jump rope
- Two or more players

20. **Simple Tag (aerobic)**—"It" tries to tag another player. When a player is tagged, he must call out "I'm it!" and the game continues.

**Variations**

- Shadow tag—a player is tagged when "it" crosses their shadow
- Towel tag—"it" tags people by hitting them below the waist with a towel
- Poison tag—"it" must place his hand on the spot where he was tagged.
- Equipment for Towel tag: a towel
- Three or more players

21. **Safe Tag (aerobic, muscular fitness)**—The game is played like simple tag except when a player is in a certain position he is safe and cannot be tagged. The type of safe position is designated before the game. A safe position could be walking like an animal, seal, crab, rabbit, etc., or exercises such as jumping jacks, push-ups, sit-ups, etc.

- Equipment: none
- Three or more players

22. **Birdie Dunk (striking)**—This game is basketball played with a shuttlecock and badminton racquet or cardboard, instead of a basketball. The object of the game is to hit the shuttlecock to teammates until one is in position to hit the "birdie" into a basket. A player may pass to himself. Hands cannot touch the birdie (penalty is loss of possession.) If the birdie touches the floor, it is awarded to the team playing defense. Baskets may be pails set at any height.
    - Equipment: badminton racquet
    - Two or more players

23. **Boccie (throwing / rolling)**—This is a traditional Italian game similar to bowling, played on a lawn or other surface outdoors. Players roll or throw a ball toward a target. The ball nearest the target wins. All ages can play together.
    - Equipment: ball, target
    - Two or more players

24. **Frisbee Golf (throwing)**—A golf course is laid out with "pins" to hit. The "pins" can be trees, tin cans, pails, etc. Each player attempts to throw his Frisbee at the first pin. The Frisbee must be thrown from the spot where it has landed on the ground. Players move from pin to pin until the course is completed. Each player's score is the number of throws needed to complete the course.
    - Equipment: Frisbee, "pins"
    - Two or more players

25. **Miniature Golf Croquet (striking)**—Set up a miniature golf course using croquet wicket hoops. Place obstacles (tree, pail, board, etc.) around the course. Each player takes a turn hitting his ball. Each player's score is the number of hits needed to complete the course.
    - Equipment: croquet wicket hoops; croquet mallets and balls, or miniature golf clubs and golf balls
    - Two or more players

26. **Run For Your Life (aerobic)**—A home base is selected (it can be a tree, pail, etc.) Player A covers her eyes and counts to 50 while the other players hide. Player A then hunts for the players in hiding. When player A finds someone she shouts, "run for your life!" Everyone else runs as fast as they can and tries to get back to home. Player A tries to tag them before they can reach home base.
    - Equipment: none
    - Two or more players

27. **Red Rover (aerobic)**—Children line up on one edge of the lawn. One person is "it." "It" announces, "Red Rover, Red Rover, whoever is wearing ("it" says a color) come over." The players who are wearing that color must cross to the other side of the yard without being touched by "it." Those who are caught become a tagger. "It" then calls a different color until all children have crossed over.
    - Equipment: none
    - Three or more players

28. **Two Man Kickball (aerobic)**—Set two bases 20 to 50 feet apart depending upon the age of players (20 feet apart for the younger players, and 30 feet apart for the older players.) The pitcher rolls the ball

to the kicker. The kicker kicks the ball and runs from home to first base as many times as he can before the pitcher can tag one of the bases with the ball. The score is equal to the number of bases the runner touched before the pitcher tags a base while holding the ball. They then switch places and the pitcher becomes the kicker. There is no out of bounds so any kick is a legal kick. The person with the highest score after 5 innings wins.

**Variation:** Have two people play defense, but each person keeps separate totals of their points.

- Equipment: kickball
- Three or more players

29. **Line Pass Tag (aerobic)**—Draw boxes and circles on the driveway so that all the lines are connected. Divide into two teams. Have one foam ball for every four players. A tagging team is designated. All players must run on the lines. The team with the ball or balls tries to tag the opposing team by touching the opponent with the ball held in your hand. The person without the ball cannot run. The person without the ball can run. Taggers pass the ball back and forth to get into position to tag an opponent. When an opponent is tagged, he leaves the game. If the tagging team drops a passed ball, a player may re-enter the game. When a pass is dropped, they lose possession of the ball and the other team becomes the taggers. Game ends when one team has been eliminated.

- Equipment: foam balls
- Four or more players

30. **Soccer Steal (aerobic)**—A playing area is marked off (approximately 30 x 30 feet). One player is designated the stealer. All other players have a soccer ball. At the start of the game, players dribble the ball with their feet and the stealer attempts to steal a soccer ball using only his feet. The person who loses their ball becomes the new stealer. A larger group can have more stealers.

- Equipment: soccer balls
- Three or more players

31. **Flashlight Tag (aerobic)**—The game is played at night in a yard or park. The person who is "it" counts aloud to 50 while the others hide. Armed with a flashlight, "it" searches for the others (the flashlight must stay on and can not be covered.) If "it" spots a person, he must get close enough to identify the person and call out his or her name. The person is then caught. You can choose a variation of what happens next: the person caught can become the next "it," or go to jail. In jail, the person will wait until all are caught or the person may be freed from jail if tagged by another teammate.

- Equipment: none
- Three or more players

32. **Hang Time**—One player throws or kicks a ball into the air. The second player uses a stopwatch to time how long the ball is aloft (time starts when the ball leaves the foot or hand, and stops when the ball touches the ground.) Longest hang time wins.

- Equipment: ball, stopwatch
- Two or more players

# SNOW GAMES

Parents should be aware of safety precautions for winter activities (see pages 32–33). Be sure that children have appropriate boots and gloves to protect from frostbite.

1. **Snow Shoveling (aerobic, upper body muscles)**—Our children love to build snow forts. Give them a junior-size, plastic shovel to reduce the injury potential. You can tell them to take the snow off the driveway to build the fort in the yard—this way, they will have fun without even knowing they are doing a chore! Appropriate for ALL ages.
   - Equipment: junior-size snow shovels
   - One or more players

2. **Designs In the Snow (aerobic, lower body muscles)**—Fresh snow is like a magnet to children. Have them make paths or create designs in the snow by shuffling their feet.
   - Equipment: junior-size snow shovels
   - One or more players

3. **Snow Tag (excellent aerobics)**—Play Freeze Tag in the snow. Tag a person by touching him or hitting him with a snowball. (No hitting in the face!) Playing tag using cross-country skis (with no poles) or snow shoes will give an opportunity to practice these sport skills, too.
   - Equipment: optional cross-country skis, snow shoes
   - Three or more players

4. **Sled Dog Races (aerobic)**—Have sprint races while pulling sleds. Add people or objects to the sled. Set up a course, race uphill, and slide downhill to the finish line.
   - Equipment: sleds
   - Two or more players

5. **Snow Baseball (aerobic, batting)**—Use a plastic bat and ball. Be sure to paint the ball a bright color so you can spot it in the snow.
   - Equipment: plastic bat and ball
   - Two or more players

6. **Snow Soccer (aerobic, soccer skills)**—The snow makes the play slower, but kicking is a real challenge!
   - Equipment: soccer ball
   - Two or more players

7. **Snow Shoe or Cross-Country Ski Races (aerobic)**—Have the children make snow shoes out of plastic pail lids. Have a race around, uphill, and downhill.
   - Equipment: plastic pail lids (or snowshoes)
   - Two or more players

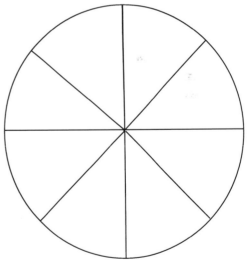

8. **Pie In The Snow (aerobic)**—In fresh snow, stomp down the snow in the shape of a round pie, approximately 20 feet in diameter; form trails that divide the "pie" into eight pieces. Play regular

Tag or Freeze Tag; players can only run on the trails. The center of the pie can be designated as a safe zone, but only one person is allowed on the safe zone at a time (if a new person enters the safe zone, the person there must leave).

- Equipment: none
- Three or more players

9. **Snow Badminton (aerobic, striking)**—Play badminton in the snow. Place the net higher to allow more time to move to the birdie.
   - Equipment: badminton equipment
   - Two or more players

## TRAMPOLINE GAMES

Backyard trampolines have become very popular. They are great for building coordination and aerobic endurance.

**A warning:** I do not recommend using a trampoline unless it has a mesh cage around it. The cage will help prevent children from falling off and getting hurt. I also suggest you limit the number of children on the trampoline at one time to four.

**A note:** Trampolines have different weight restrictions depending on the size and manufacturer. The total weight of the children should not exceed the manufacturer's weight limit.

1. **Popcorn**—Place 4 to 8 Nerf balls or tennis balls on the trampoline. The children hop around to get the balls to move. Play stops when a child is touched by a ball, and play begins again with one less child. Continue until only one child is left.
2. **War**—All players stand on the trampoline. On the command 1–2–3, all players drop to the trampoline in a sitting position and rebound back to a standing position. When a player does not rebound to a standing position, he is eliminated. Play continues until one player is left.
3. **Blind Tiger**—One person is "it." "It" closes his eyes and is in the middle of the trampoline on his hands and knees. On the command, "it" crawls around and tries to tag other players. Other players have their eyes open and are free to be in constant motion to stay away from "it."

## Backyard Equipment

If you are interested in installing a few simple pieces of equipment to increase the range of games you can play in your backyard, I have listed a few items below that can be purchased and installed.

**Fireman pole**—Builds upper body strength. Bolt an iron pipe (aprox. 2" diameter) to a tree, treehouse, or swing set. Children can have races going up the treehouse and down the pole, or up the pole and down the ladder.

**Climbing rope**—Builds upper body strength. A rope 1 inch in diameter can be hung from a tree. Challenge your child to climb to the top of the rope without using his or her feet. If the rope will be used for swinging, tie a loop to the bottom of the rope for a foothold (make sure the loop is smaller than a child's head.) No rules, just hours of fun swinging!

**Large inner tube**—The larger the tube, the heavier the child can be. Use the giant tube like a mini-tramp to jump on. A child can do stunts, including knee drops and seat drops.

You can also play War (two people stand on the tube and try to bounce each other off. No pushing or body contact is allowed. This is a great balance game.)

We have had an inner tube in the family for over 30 years and never had an injury! Playing on the inner tube has been everyone's favorite summer activity, hands down. **Hint:** to find a large enough tube, call a snow, hill, or river tubing business, or a local tire supplier for a tractor tire.

**Swing set**—Add a trapeze bar and rings to a regular swing to help develop upper body strength. (Place mats under the rings to cover the cement floor or hard surface, to avoid injury in case your child falls.)

**Jungle gym**—Inexpensive PVC pipe from a hardware store can be used to fashion a jungle gym in the basement or outdoors. Younger children can have hours of fun!

## INDOOR GAMES

| Activity | Grade | Number of Players | Aerobics | Muscle Endurance | Coordination | Balance | Dodging | Movement | Throwing | Catching | Shooting | Striking | Kicking |
|---|---|---|---|---|---|---|---|---|---|---|---|---|---|
| **1.** Simon Says | K–3 | 2+ | X | X | | | | X | | | | | |
| **2.** Follow the Leader | K–6 | 2+ | X | X | | | | X | | | | | |
| **3.** Forty Ways to Get There | K–4 | 2+ | | | X | | | X | | | | | |
| **4.** Four Square | 1–up | 2+ | | | X | | | | | | | X | |
| **5.** Hopscotch | K–5 | 2+ | | X | X | X | | X | | | | | |
| **6.** Balloon Volleyball | K–3 | 2+ | | | X | | | | | | | X | |
| **7.** Indoor Mini-Basketball | K–up | 1+ | | | | | | | | | X | | |
| **8.** Pin Guard | K–up | 2+ | | | X | | | | X | | | | |
| **9.** Dodgeball | K–up | 2+ | X | | | | X | X | X | | | | |
| **10.** Keep Away | K–up | 3+ | X | | | | | | X | | | | |
| **11.** Blanket Toss | K–3 | 2+ | | | X | | | | | | | | |
| **12.** Flashlight Tag | K–up | 3+ | | X | | | | X | | | | | |
| **13.** Tiger Tails | K–up | 2+ | X | | X | | X | | | | | | |
| **14.** Fox and Rabbit | K–6 | 4+ | X | | X | | | | X | X | | | |
| **15.** Floor Tennis | 1–5 | 2+ | | | X | | | | | | | X | |

| Activity | Grade | Number of Players | Aerobics | Muscle Endurance | Coordination | Balance | Dodging | Movement | Throwing | Catching | Shooting | Striking | Kicking |
|---|---|---|---|---|---|---|---|---|---|---|---|---|---|
| 16. Badminiature | 1–5 | 2+ | | | X | | | | | | | X | |
| 17. Beanbag Toss | 1+ | 1+ | | | X | | | | X | | X | | |
| 18. Sardines | K–up | 3+ | | | | | | | | | | | |
| 19. Obstacle Course | K–up | 1+ | X | X | X | | | | | | | | |
| 20. Can Race | 1–up | 2+ | X | X | X | X | | | | | | | |
| 21. Wild Ball | 1–up | 2+ | X | X | X | | | | | | | | |
| 22. Fool Ball | 2–up | 3+ | | | X | | | | X | X | | X | |
| 23. Musical Balloons | K–up | 4+ | | | X | | | | | X | | | |
| 24. Car | K–up | 3+ | X | | | | X | | | | | | |
| 25. Hack Four Square | 1–up | 2+ | | | X | | | | | | | X | |

## OUTDOOR GAMES

| Activity | Grade | Number of Players | Aerobics | Muscle Endurance | Coordination | Balance | Dodging | Movement | Throwing | Catching | Shooting | Striking | Kicking |
|---|---|---|---|---|---|---|---|---|---|---|---|---|---|
| 1. Anti-I-Over | 1–up | 2 + | | | | | | | X | X | | | |
| 2. 500 Baseball | 2–up | 3 + | | | | | | | X | X | | | |
| 3. Home Run Baseball | 1–up | 2 + | X | | | | | | X | X | | X | |
| 4. Kickball | 1–up | 2 + | X | | | | | | X | X | | | X |
| 5. Speedy Soccer | 1–up | 2 + | X | X | X | | | | | | | | X |
| 6. Newcomb Volleyball | K–4 | 2 + | | | X | | | | X | X | | X | |
| 7. Football Punt and Catch | 3–up | 2 + | | X | | | | | | X | | | X |
| 8. Frisbee Football | 1–up | 4 + | X | | | | | | X | X | | | |
| 9. Kid's Handball | 3–up | 2–4 | X | | X | | | | | | | X | |
| 10. Lightning Basketball | K–up | 2 + | X | | | | | | | | X | | |

| Activity | Grade | Number of Players | Aerobics | Muscle Endurance | Coordination | Balance | Dodging | Movement | Throwing | Catching | Shooting | Striking | Kicking |
|---|---|---|---|---|---|---|---|---|---|---|---|---|---|
| **11.** Deck Tennis | 3–up | 2–4 | X | | X | | | | X | X | | | |
| **12.** Tug of War | K–up | 2 + | | X | | | | | | | | | |
| **13.** Cops and Robbers | K–up | 4 + | X | | | | | | | | | | |
| **14.** Capture the Flag | K–up | 4 + | X | | | | | | | | | | |
| **15.** Hide and Seek | K–up | 2 + | X | | | | | | | | | | |
| **16.** Freeze Tag | K–up | 4 + | X | | | | | | | | | | |
| **17.** Blob Tag | K–up | 4 + | X | | | | | | | | | | |
| **18.** Marco Polo Tag | K–up | 3 + | X | | X | | | | | | | | |
| **19.** Snake Catcher | K–4 | 3 + | X | | X | | | | | | | | |
| **20.** Simple Tag | K–up | 3 + | X | | | | | | | | | | |
| **21.** Safe Tag | K–up | 3 + | X | | | | | | | | | | |
| **22.** Birdie Dunk | K–up | 2 + | X | | X | | | | | | | X | |
| **23.** Boccie Ball | K–up | 2 + | | | | | | | X | | | | |
| **24.** Frisbee Golf | 1+2 | 2+ | | | | | | | X | | | | |
| **25.** Miniature Golf Croquet | 1+ | 2+ | | | | | | | | | | X | |
| **26.** Run For Your Life | K–up | 2+ | X | | | | | | X | X | | | |
| **27.** Red Rover | K–up | 4+ | X | | | | X | X | | | | | |
| **28.** Two Man Kickball | K–up | 2+ | X | | | | | | | | | | X |
| **29.** Line Pass Tag | K–up | 4+ | X | | | | | | | | | | |
| **30.** Soccer Steal | K–up | 3+ | X | | | | | | | | | | X |
| **31.** Flashlight Tag | K–up | 3+ | | | | | | X | | | | | |
| **32.** Hang Time | 1–up | 2+ | | X | | | | | X | X | | | |

# SNOW GAMES

| Activity | Grade | Number of Players | Aerobics | Muscle Endurance | Coordination | Balance | Dodging | Movement | Throwing | Catching | Shooting | Striking | Kicking |
|---|---|---|---|---|---|---|---|---|---|---|---|---|---|
| **1.** Snow Shoveling | K–up | 1 + | X | X | | | | | | | | | |
| **2.** Designs in the Snow | K–up | 1 + | X | | | | | | | | | | |
| **3.** Snow Tag | K–up | 3 + | X | | | | | | | | | | |
| **4.** Sled Dog Races | K–up | 2 + | X | | | | | | | | | | |
| **5.** Snow Baseball | 1–up | 2 + | X | | | | | | X | X | | X | |
| **6.** Snow Soccer | 1–up | 2 + | X | | | | | | | | | | X |
| **7.** Snow Shoe Cross-Country Ski Races | K–up | 2 + | X | | X | X | | | | | | | |
| **8.** Pie in the Snow | K–up | 3 + | X | | | | | | | | | | |
| **9.** Snow Badminton | 1–up | 2 + | X | | X | | | | | | | X | |

# Fitness Tests

5

## YOU MAY BE WONDERING . . .

How fit is my child? How do I know what is a healthy fitness "level?" One way to answer this question is to give a formal test.

◇◇◇◇◇◇◇◇◇◇◇◇◇◇◇◇◇◇◇◇◇◇◇◇◇◇◇◇◇◇◇◇◇◇◇◇◇◇◇◇◇◇◇◇◇◇◇◇◇◇

**Public schools typically** give children the following tests:
- sit-ups, push-ups, and pull-ups—to test muscular endurance and strength
- 1-mile run/walk—to test the child's aerobic capacity

◇◇◇◇◇◇◇◇◇◇◇◇◇◇◇◇◇◇◇◇◇◇◇◇◇◇◇◇◇◇◇◇◇◇◇◇◇◇◇◇◇◇◇◇◇◇◇◇◇◇

To assist you in objectively determining the fitness level of your child, I have included tests and charts that outline the recommended minimal fitness level your child should attain.

Each family member should take these tests. Afterwards, as a family, you can discuss how each individual ranks on the charts included.

Below, I describe the two different types of tests offered in schools: The Fitnessgram, and the Presidential Fitness Test. In my opinion, the Fitnessgram tests are the best, but I have also included the Presidential Fitness Test because it is one that parents probably remember from their school days. It is up to you to decide which set of tests to take.

## FITNESSGRAM BATTERY OF TESTS

Fitnessgram was created in 1982 by The Cooper Institute to provide an easy way for physical education teachers to report students' fitness levels to their parents. Dr. Kenneth Cooper, founder of the Cooper Institute, is recognized by many as the leader of the international physical fitness movement and credited with motivating people to exercise in pursuit of good health. Today, the Fitnessgram tests are mandatory in some states for public school children (www.fitnessgram.net).

With the Fitnessgram program, students are tested in these areas:

- cardiovascular fitness
- muscle strength
- muscular endurance
- flexibility
- body composition

| Body Mass Index (BMI) | Equipment | Description |
| --- | --- | --- |
| Body mass index is a measurement of body fat based on the height and weight of the person.<br><br>**Note:** A test called a "skin fold caliper test" is also used to measure body fat. Although the skin fold caliper test is more accurate, it is harder to administer. | None (Internet access) | Measure the height and weight of the child. Then, go to one of the websites below and follow the instructions. BMI will be automatically calculated, and a report can be printed.<br><br>- http://www.cdc.gov/nccdphp/dnpa/bmi/<br>- http://www.kidsnutrition.org/bodycomp/bmiz2.html<br>- www.halls.md/ideal-weight/body.html. This site will calculate your ideal body weight. |

Scores are evaluated against standards set in the Healthy Fitness Zones, which indicate the level of fitness necessary for health. To be considered healthy, the child's score must be within the healthy fitness zone on all six tests.

I believe the Fitnessgram Test is more effective than any other physical fitness test for three reasons. First, it compares scores to carefully researched and developed health standards rather than to national averages. Second, it emphasizes measures of health-related physical fitness instead of sports-related skills. Third, it goes beyond mere measurement to recommend individualized physical activity programs that will help students improve (Fitnessgram, 1999).

# A TEST BASED ON THE FITNESSGRAM ASSESSMENT

Below is a summary chart of some of the key tests in the Fitnessgram assessment. To save time, I have included only those tests which I believe to be most effective in fully determining your child's fitness level. I have included a description of each fitness test so you can administer them yourself. I have also included blank charts for you to fill in the results yourself.

| Fitness Area | Test | Description |
|---|---|---|
| Aerobic capacity | 1-Mile Run/Walk | Walk or run for 1 mile as fast as possible. |
| Abdominal muscle strength and endurance | Curl-Up Test | Complete as many curl-ups as possible up to 75. |
| Trunk extensor flexibility | Trunk Lift | Lift the upper body 12 inches off the floor using the muscles of the back. The lift must be held long enough so the distance of the upper body from the floor can be measured. |
| Upper body strength and endurance | Push-up | Complete as many push-ups as possible at a specific pace of one every 3 seconds. |
| Flexibility (of the lower back and posterior thigh) | Sit and Reach Test | The individual sits with legs straight in front of them and extends their arms as far as possible. |
| Body composition | Body Mass Index | This is a mathematical calculation that provides an estimate of body fat, and risk of becoming overweight, through the measure of weight relative to height. |

## TESTS
## 1-Mile Run/Walk

This test measures the aerobic capacity of the heart and lungs. In this test, you will time how long it takes to run or walk for 1 mile. Measure the length of 1 mile with a car or bicycle. Or, if you are conducting the test at a 400-meter track, 1 mile is 4 laps plus 10 yards.

## EQUIPMENT

Pencil, paper, stopwatch

## DESCRIPTION

Run or walk at an even pace, without stopping. Note: It is acceptable to run with intermittent walking breaks if a running pace cannot be maintained.

## Curl-up Test

8. Curl up test

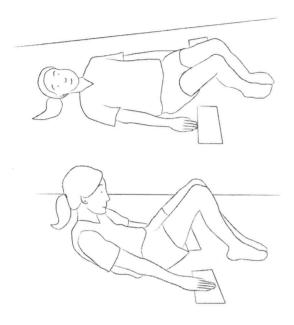

This test measures the strength and endurance of the abdominal muscles. The students complete as many curl-ups as they can. The curl-up has been selected because, unlike a regular sit-up, it does not involve the assistance of the hip flexor muscles.

### EQUIPMENT

Tape, piece of 8.5" x 11" paper, gym mat or carpeting, piece of cardboard 4.5 x 8.5".

Two people are needed to conduct this test.

### DESCRIPTION:

Partner A lies on the mat, face up, with knees bent at approximately 140 degrees. Partner B should be positioned near the knees. A piece of paper should be under the head. Partner B tapes the piece of cardboard to the mat where it just touches the fingertips of Partner A (the long side of the cardboard should touch the fingertips.) Partner A extends the arms towards the feet, palms facing down, and slowly lifts up the trunk of the body until the fingers have moved 4.5", across the width of the cardboard. Partner A then curls back down until the head returns to the mat. It will be clear that the head has returned to the mat because the paper will move and wrinkle when the head touches it. Partner B should count each correctly done curl-up. A curl-up should only be counted if the fingers move 4½ inches, across the entire width of the cardboard.

Stop at 75 curl-ups, or when the individual cannot complete one curl-up every 3 seconds.

## Trunk Lift Test

This test measures the strength and flexibility of the muscles in the lower back.

6. Trunk lift

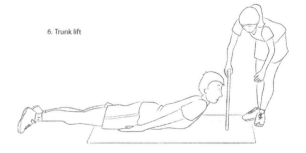

### EQUIPMENT:

Ruler or piece of paper, marked at 6", 9", and 12" tape. Two people are needed to conduct this test.

### DESCRIPTION:

Partner A begins lying face down with the hands under the hips. Partner B holds the ruler and sits at the head of Partner A. Place a piece of tape on the floor directly below Partner A's eyes. Partner A lifts the upper body off the floor in a slow, controlled movement to a maximum of 12 inches. The eyes should focus on the tape and the head should remain in line with the spine. Partner A will hold this position until Partner B can measure the distance from the mat to the chin.

## Push-up Test

This test measures the strength and endurance of the muscles in the upper body, including the muscles of the arms, shoulder, upper back, and chest.

### EQUIPMENT:

None

### DESCRIPTION:

Begin face-down on the floor with palms slightly wider than the shoulders and legs extended, with feet together. Complete as many push-ups as possible, beginning each push-up with a 90-degree bend in the elbows and finishing with the arms fully extended and the body straight from toes to shoulders. Repeat at a rate of one push-up per 3 seconds.

The test ends when the individual being tested: (1) stops to rest; (2) does not maintain a 90-degree angle when bending elbows; (3) does not maintain correct body position; (4) does not extend arms fully.

## Modified Push-up Test: The Knee Push-up

If your child is unable to do a regular push-up, you can test them with the knee push-up.

### DESCRIPTION

Begin face down on the floor with palms slightly wider than the shoulders and legs together. Bend the knees to the floor and keep the back straight. Lower the body until the elbows are bent at a 90-degree angle. The knees should remain bent during the push-ups. Do as many as possible in 1 minute. The test ends if the individual being tested: (1) stops to rest; (2) does not maintain a 90-degree angle when bending elbows; (3) does not maintain correct body position; (4) does not extend arms fully.

## Sit and Reach Test

7. Sit and reach test

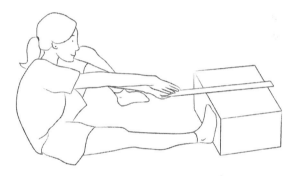

This test measures the flexibility of the hamstring muscles. Both the right and left sides of the body are tested separately.

### EQUIPMENT:

Ruler, tape. This test should be conducted at the bottom of a staircase.

### DESCRIPTION:

Tape a ruler to the top of the bottom step of a staircase. The 9-inch mark should be flush with the edge of the step, with the lower numbers overhanging the edge of the step.

Remove the shoes. Sit on the floor with the right foot fully extended and flat against the stair. The left leg is bent so that the bottom of the left foot is pressed to the back of the right knee. Place one hand on top of the other, palms down, and extend the arms. Reach as far forward as possible and hold the position for approximately 2 seconds, so the length of the extension can be read on the ruler. After one side is measured, switch legs and repeat the test.

## READING THE RESULTS:
## STANDARDS FOR HEALTHY FITNESS LEVELS

These standards represent the level of fitness necessary for health. To be considered healthy, the child's score must be within the healthy fitness zone on all six tests.

## Males

| Age | 1-mile run Min:sec | Body Mass Index | Curl-up # completed | Trunk Lift inches | Push-up* # completed | Sit and Reach inches |
|---|---|---|---|---|---|---|
| 5 | | 20–14.7 | 2–10 | 6–12 | 3–8 | 8 |
| 6 | | 20–14.7 | 2–10 | 6–12 | 3–8 | 8 |
| 7 | | 20–14.9 | 4–14 | 6–12 | 4–10 | 8 |
| 8 | | 20–15.1 | 6–20 | 6–12 | 5–13 | 8 |
| 9 | | 20–13.7 | 9–24 | 6–12 | 6–15 | 8 |
| 10 | 11:30–9:00 | 21–14 | 12–24 | 9–12 | 7–20 | 8 |
| 11 | 11:00–8:30 | 21–14.3 | 15–28 | 9–12 | 8–20 | 8 |
| 12 | 10:30–8:00 | 22–14.6 | 18–36 | 9–12 | 10–20 | 8 |
| 13 | 10:00–7:30 | 23–15.1 | 21–40 | 9–12 | 12–25 | 8 |
| 14 | 9:30–7:00 | 24.5–15.6 | 24–45 | 9–12 | 14–30 | 8 |
| 15 | 9:00–7:00 | 25–16.2 | 24–47 | 9–12 | 16–35 | 8 |
| 16 | 8:30–7:00 | 26.5–16.6 | 24–47 | 9–12 | 18–35 | 8 |
| 17 | 8:30–7:00 | 27–17.3 | 24–47 | 9–12 | 18–35 | 8 |
| 17+ | 8:30–7:00 | 27.8–17.8 | 24–47 | 9–12 | 18–35 | 8 |

**A note:** When looking at the results for the 1-mile run/walk and BMI, the smaller numbers are better. For the remaining four tests, the larger numbers are better.

# Females

| Age | 1-mile run Min:sec | Body Mass Index | Curl-up # completed | Trunk Lift inches | Push-up/ Modified Push-up # completed | Sit and Reach inches |
|---|---|---|---|---|---|---|
| 5 | | 21–16.2 | 2–10 | 6–12 | 3–8 | 9 |
| 6 | | 21–16.2 | 2–10 | 6–12 | 3–8 | 9 |
| 7 | | 22–16.2 | 4–14 | 6–12 | 4–10 | 9 |
| 8 | | 22–16.2 | 6–20 | 6–12 | 5–13 | 9 |
| 9 | | 23–13.5 | 9–22 | 6–12 | 6–15 | 9 |
| 10 | 12:30–9:30 | 23.5–13.7 | 12–26 | 9–12 | 7–15 | 9 |
| 11 | 12:00–9:00 | 24–14 | 15–29 | 9–12 | 7–15 | 10 |
| 12 | 12:00–9:00 | 24.5–14.5 | 18–32 | 9–12 | 7–15 | 10 |
| 13 | 11:30–9:00 | 24.5–14.9 | 18–32 | 9–12 | 7–15 | 10 |
| 14 | 11:00–8:30 | 25–15.4 | 18–32 | 9–12 | 7–15 | 10 |
| 15 | 10:30–8:00 | 25–16 | 18–35 | 9–12 | 7–15 | 12 |
| 16 | 10:00–8:00 | 25–16.4 | 18–35 | 9–12 | 7–15 | 12 |
| 17 | 10:00–8:00 | 26–16.8 | 18–35 | 9–12 | 7–15 | 12 |
| 17+ | 10:00–8:00 | 27.3–17.2 | 18–35 | 9–12 | 7–15 | 12 |

Copyrighted 2006 by the Cooper Institute, Dallas Texas

For parents interested in knowing how they measure up (when they complete as many push-ups as possible with no more than a 3 second pause between) see below.

| | Average | Excellent |
|---|---|---|
| Men ages 30–39 | 25–35 | 33–45 |
| Women ages 30–39 (modified push-up) | 15–25 | 25–40 |

The Official YMCA Physical Fitness Handbook, 1975

# LAB: FITNESS TESTS

Name: _____ Age: _____

## Instructions:

Administer the fitness tests to your child as described and record the results on the chart below.

Afterwards, look at the results and answer:

♦ Were the child's scores higher than the scores recommended for a minimal level of fitness?

♦ Did your child excel in any areas?

♦ Is your child weak in any areas?

♦ Then, sit down with your child and evaluate the results together. You can discuss ways in which he or she can improve. If you have taken the test yourself, you can also discuss your own plans for getting more fit.

| | Mile Run (time) | BMI (index) | Curl-up (#completed) | Trunk Lift (inches) | Push-up (#completed) | Bent Arm Hang (seconds) | Sit & Reach (inches) | Knee Push-ups (#completed) |
|---|---|---|---|---|---|---|---|---|
| **Your score** | | | | | | | | |
| **Minimum score to be fit** | | | | | | | | |
| **Did you meet the minimum score?** | Yes<br>No | Yes<br>No | Yes<br>No | Yes<br>No | Yes<br>No | Yes<br>No | Yes<br>No | Yes<br>No |

## Supplemental Test

Listed below are other tests that have been used in public schools for decades. The Fitnessgram test is gaining in popularity and is slowly replacing these tests. However, these tests can still be helpful in assessing the fitness of your child, and you may chose to use them if you like.

### FLEXED-ARM HANG TEST

This test has been used for years in public schools to measure the strength and endurance of the muscles of the arms, shoulders, upper chest, and back. To be at a minimal level of fitness, results should meet or exceed the score listed below.

## Equipment:
Chin-up bar

## Description

Grasp the bar with both hands, with the palms facing outward. The feet must not touch the ground and the body should not swing. Raise the body until the chin is level with the top of the bar. Hold this position as long as possible. The score is calculated based on the number of seconds the individual can hang with their chin above the bar.

Compare the resulting score to the average scores listed below.

| Age | Girls Seconds | Boys Seconds |
|---|---|---|
| 5 | 5 | 5 |
| 6 | 5 | 5 |
| 7 | 5 | 5 |
| 8 | 8 | 10 |
| 9 | 8 | 10 |
| 10 | 8 | 10 |
| 11 | 8 | 10 |
| 12 | 8 | 10 |
| 13 | 12 | 10 |
| 14 | 12 | 15 |
| 15 | 12 | 25 |
| 16 | 12 | 25 |
| 17 | 12 | 25 |

*Kid Fitness* by Dr. Kenneth H. Cooper. Bantam Books, 1991, pp 104–5.

## PRESIDENT'S CHALLENGE TEST

This is the test most parents will remember taking in school. At the end of the President's Challenge, the students who scored above the eighty-fifth percentile in all the tests received an award, the Presidential Physical Fitness Award.

This test is not very helpful for parents who are trying to determine how healthy their child is because its rankings are based on how many children the individual out-performed, and this type of ranking does not present a medical performance level of health. For this reason, I do not recommend using the President's Challenge test, but I am including it here in case you have a motivated child who would like a challenge.

Please visit the internet for further details at www.presidentschallenge.org/educators/program_details/physical_fitness_test.aspx.

## FAMILY FITNESS CHALLENGE

Taking a fitness test together as a family can be fun! It can also be a great way to communicate to your children that taking your own health seriously is important, too. This test has "modifications" built in, so it will be appropriate for all ages and skill levels. The test measures a variety of components of fitness.

The scoring system in the Family Fitness Challenge is based on a decathlon scoring system. With this system, any child can earn an award if they work toward it.

Details on how to administer and perform all of these tests, except for jump rope and the 50-yard dash (which are self-explanatory,) are given earlier in this chapter, so directions are not repeated here.

| Tests | Measures What |
|-------|---------------|
| Sit and Reach | Flexibility fitness |
| 1-Mile Run walk | Aerobic fitness |
|  | Heart/lungs |
| Sit-ups | Muscle fitness |
|  | Abdominal strength |
| Flexed-Arm Hang | Muscle fitness |
|  | Arm strength |
| Jump Rope | Coordination |
| 50-Yard Dash | Speed |

| Grade | Points needed to earn an award |
|-------|--------------------------------|
| 1 | 25 |
| 2 | 30 |
| 3 | 33 |
| 4 | 35 |
| 5 | 40 |
| 6 | 43 |
| 7 | 45 |
| 8 | 47 |
| 9 | 50 |
| 10 | 52 |
| 11 | 54 |
| 12 | 55 |

## 1-Mile Run walk

| Score in minutes | Points |
|---|---|
| 10:15–+ | .5 |
| 10:01–10:14 | 1 |
| 9:45–10:00 | 2 |
| 9:31–9:44 | 2.5 |
| 9:15–9:30 | 3 |
| 9:01–9:14 | 3.5 |
| 8:31–9:00 | 4 |
| 8:15–8:30 | 5 |
| 8:01–8:14 | 5.5 |
| 7:45–8:00 | 6 |
| 7:31–7:44 | 6.5 |
| 7:15–7:30 | 7 |
| 7:01–7:14 | 7.5 |
| 6:45—7:00 | 8 |
| 6:31—6:44 | 8.5 |
| 6:15—6:30 | 9 |
| 6:01—6:14 | 9.5 |
| 6:00—+ | 10 |

## Flexed-Arm Hang

| Score in seconds | Points |
|---|---|
| 1–2 | 1 |
| 3–6 | 2 |
| 7–14 | 3 |
| 15–23 | 4 |
| 24–30 | 5 |
| 31–37 | 6 |
| 38–44 | 7 |
| 45–52 | 8 |
| 53–59 | 9 |
| 60–+ | 10 |
| 60–+ | 10 |

## Sit-ups

| Score | Points |
|---|---|
| 1–10 | .5 |
| 11–19 | 1 |
| 20–24 | 2 |
| 25–29 | 3 |
| 30–34 | 4 |
| 35–39 | 5 |
| 40–44 | 6 |
| 45–49 | 7 |
| 50–54 | 8 |
| 55–59 | 9 |
| 60–+ | 10 |

## 50-Yard Dash

| Score in seconds | Points |
|---|---|
| 10.1–+ | 1 |
| 9.6–10.0 | 2 |
| 9.1–9.5 | 3 |
| 8.6–9.0 | 4 |
| 8.1–8.5 | 5 |
| 7.6–8.0 | 6 |
| 7.1–7.5 | 7 |
| 6.6–7.0 | 8 |
| 6.1–6.5 | 9 |
| 6.0–+ | 10 |

## Jump Rope in 30 Seconds

| Score in number of jumps | Points |
|---|---|
| 1–4 | .5 |
| 5–9 | 1 |
| 10–14 | 1.5 |
| 15–19 | 2 |
| 20–24 | 2.5 |
| 25–29 | 3 |
| 30–34 | 3.5 |
| 35–39 | 4 |
| 40–44 | 4.5 |
| 45–49 | 5 |
| 50–54 | 5.5 |
| 55–59 | 6 |
| 60–64 | 6.5 |
| 65–69 | 7 |
| 70–74 | 7.5 |
| 75–79 | 8 |
| 80–84 | 8.5 |
| 85–89 | 9 |
| 90–94 | 9.5 |
| 95-+ | 10 |

## Sit and Reach

| Score in inches | Points |
|---|---|
| 1 | .5 |
| 2 | 1 |
| 3 | 1.5 |
| 4 | 2 |
| 5 | 2.5 |
| 6 | 3 |
| 7 | 3.5 |
| 8 | 4 |
| 9 | 4.5 |
| 10 | 5 |
| 11 | 5.5 |
| 12 | 6 |
| 13 | 6.5 |
| 14 | 7 |
| 15 | 7.5 |
| 16 | 8 |
| 17 | 8.5 |
| 18 | 9 |
| 19 | 9.5 |
| 20-+ | 10 |

**Note:** The student counts how many times they jump the rope in 30 seconds.

## One final note . . .

Don't forget why you are giving your child these tests: these scores indicate how healthy he or she is, and how prepared he or she is to participate in strenuous physical activity. If your child does not meet these minimal requirements, he or she will be more susceptible to injury and to health problems, so you should be sure to work further on problem areas.

# Lesson Plans

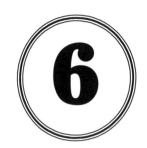

**BODY MOVEMENT FUNDAMENTALS UNIT**

**BALL SKILLS UNIT**

**TUMBLING AND GYMNASTICS UNIT**

**SWIMMING UNIT**

**RHYTHM AND DANCE UNIT**

**LESSON PLANS**

JUST LIKE LEARNING math or any other subject, physical education begins with the basics and gradually moves on to more challenging exercises. In physical edication, the "basics" are fundamental motor skills. These must be learned in the early years of a child's life, before more complex sport skills can be learned successfully.

Do you remember how challenging it was when you first learned to skip, jump rope, or ride a bike without training wheels? We often forget that what seems easy to us now was very challenging when we were learning it for the first time. The elementary school activities below may seem easy and simple to you as an adult, but they are the building blocks for your child's motor skills and coordination, which are important for future participation in sports and more complex exercises.

The following lesson plans progress from simple to more advanced activities in each area of concentration. The areas of concentration are:

1. locomotor movement
2. ball-handling skills

3. stunts, tumbling, gymnastics
4. rhythm/dance
5. swimming

In the public school system, there is generally a focus on developing these skills in grades K through 6.

## How to Use Lesson Plans

The following lesson plans are divided into three areas: purpose, preparation, and participation.

♦ The **purpose** describes the desired skill level for the child to obtain.

♦ **Preparation** lists equipment you will need.

♦ **Participation** lists the order of skills to learn.

Each child grows and matures at his or her own rate. Some skills may come easily, and others may take longer to develop. Be aware that you may need to spend more time on some activities than others in order for your child to master the skill. At the same time, if your child finds an activity to be easy, then you can feel free to progress through the program at a faster pace.

## FOUNDATION OF BODY MOVEMENT UNIT

From the day we are born we are moving our bodies. Babies learn movement naturally, simply through doing, and they gradually progress from crawling, to walking, to running. By the time the child reaches grades K through 3, movement education begins. Movement education provides a foundation for the child's future movement exercises and sports participation. Like a baby progressing from crawling to walking, movement education should progress in a certain order so that all locomotor movements can be learned well.

## Walking, Running, and Jumping Lessons
### PURPOSE

Perform basic body locomotion movement.

### PREPARATION

Find a room or area outdoors where you and your child can work on these movements together.

### PARTICIPATION
#### Walk/Run

Ask you children the following questions to encourage him or her to complete certain movements:

**I have developed** these programs with home school families in mind; many of these activities do not require a lot of equipment or facilities and many can be done with a limited number of children. These activies are particularly useful because they will give the home school parent an understanding of which activities are appropriate for what age. From there, the home school parent can develop her own ideas.

The modified games charts (pages 59–62) will assist you in choosing the right games to build particular skills.

1. Can you walk around the room without touching objects or people?

2. How fast can you walk? How slow can you walk? (speed)

3. Can you walk forward, backward, and sideways? (direction)

4. How few steps can you take to get across the room/yard? (size)

5. How quietly can you walk? How loudly can you walk? (force)

6. Can you walk with your body very high? Very low? (heights)

7. Substitute running for all the above.

## Jumping

1. Can you jump in the air and land on two feet? (jumping)

2. Get down low (squat) and jump as high as you can.

3. Stand tall (straight) and jump as high as you can. Did you jump higher when you started down low, or up high?

5. Jump and turn in the air before landing. How far can you turn?

6. Run . . . then jump!

7. Stand still. Now, jump! Did you jump higher when you were running, or when you were standing still?

8. Jump like a kangaroo! Go forwards and backwards.

9. (Parent: tie a sting between two chairs, and progressively raise the string to see how high he or she can jump.) Jump over the string.

10. Stand still. Now jump as far forward as you can (This is called a standing broad jump. Can his distance improve with practice?

11. Move through the obstacle course! (Parent: lay small cardboard boxes on the floor 2 to 3 feet apart. Assign the student to jump over the box, in and out of the box, and around the box. As the child grows, use taller boxes.)

12. Jump on the colors! (Parent: Place colored paper squares on the floor. Call out a color sequence—for example, red, green, blue—and have your child jump onto the corresponding square. If slipping is a problem, have your child land beside the square, not on it.)

## Many Ways of Moving Lesson
### PURPOSE

Perform the movements of walking, running, jumping, skipping, hopping, sliding, galloping, and leaping.

### PREPARATION

None

### PARTICIPATION
#### Walking

1. Balance on one leg with eyes closed.

2. Walk with eyes closed.

3. Walk on heels, toes, inside and outside of the feet.

4. Lower the body while walking.

5. Raise the body while walking.

6. Walk with gliding steps, now walk with choppy steps.

7. Take long steps, short steps.

8. Walk quickly, walk slowly.

9. Walk bringing knees up high.

10. Walk and clap your hands at the same time.

11. Walk forward, walk backward.

**12.** Do the Running and Walking Lab (see chapter 7).

**Running**

**1.**

**3.** Explore different arm positions while you run. Which is the best? *

**4.** Run and stop.

**5.** Run and change directions.

**6.** Bounce as you run.

**7.** Run low, touching the ground.

**8.** Run forward, run backward.

\* Proper technique is described in the Lab "Running and Walking."

**Hopping: Hopping from one foot and landing on the same foot.**

**1.** Hop on right foot.

**2.** Hop on left foot.

**3.** Hop high, hop low.

**4.** Change directions while hopping.

**5.** Hop in place, hop ahead.

**6.** Play Hopscotch (chapter 4)

**Jumping: Jump from one or both feet and land on both feet.**

**1.** Jump and land with feet apart.

**2.** Jump and land with feet together.

**Leaping: Jump from one foot and land on the other foot.**

**1.** How high can you leap?

**2.** How far can you leap?

**3.** Leap over objects.

**Skipping: Step-hop, step-hop, swing arms and stay on the toes.**

**1.** Skip fast, skip slow.

**2.** Skip and clap.

**Sliding: Move sideways on the balls of the feet. Feet never cross.**

**1.** Slide in a direction and change directions.

**2.** Slide fast, slide slow.

**Galloping: Lead with the right foot always in front of the left foot.**

**1.** Gallop using short slides, long slides.

**2.** Gallop slow, gallop fast.

**Games**

Below are two games you can play with one child or a group of children. The parent calls out commands and the children respond.

**1. Body Alphabet:** Alone or with a partner, make the letters of the alphabet as I call them out.

**2. Animal game:** How do you think animals move? Move like the animal I call out (Parents: you can call out animals such as snake, rabbit, eagle, pony).

**3.** See chapter 4 for more games.

You can also make an outdoor slalom course. Use a stopwatch to time how long it takes for each student to run, hop, and skip around objects (objects and movements include: walk between ladder rungs, under ropes, around chairs)

## Beanbag and Movement Lesson

Beanbags are excellent for students learning to catch, because they form to the hand and do not bounce. They can be used inside and are less likely to break household items or cause personal injury. They are inexpensive and can be used for bases, goals, markers, etc. Beanbags can be made from scraps of material and filled loosely with unpopped popcorn.

## PURPOSE

1. Improve eye/hand coordination.
2. Practice tossing and catching.

## PREPARATION

One beanbag per child

## PARTICIPATION

1. Place the beanbag on your head and walk, run, hop, slide, gallop, jump, and leap. Try to keep the bag on your head as you move.
2. Toss the beanbag into the air and catch it. Toss and catch while moving.
3. Ask your child: Which body parts can you use to catch the beanbag?
4. Toss the beanbag into the air—low, medium, high.
5. Catch the beanbag low, catch it high.
6. Toss the beanbag. Clap hands and catch it.
7. Toss one beanbag with a partner.
8. Toss two beanbags at the same time.
9. Catch the beanbag with two hands, one hand.
10. Throw the beanbag from behind your back, over the shoulder, and catch it in front.
11. Toss and catch the bag with the back of your hand.
12. Toss the beanbag, do a full turn and catch.
13. Toss the beanbag, touch the floor and catch.
14. Throw the beanbag underhand, overhand, sidearm.
15. Sit down. Throw and catch the bag with a partner.
16. Toss the beanbag in various directions to make the partner move to catch it.
17. Cut a hole in a cardboard box and toss the bag through the hole.
18. Toss the beanbag into the air, clap hands, and catch it.
19. Juggle two beanbags.
20. Do the Overhand Throw Lab (chapter 7)
21. Toss the beanbag onto a specific stair step.

## GAMES

See Chapter 4
Rabbit & Fox

# Hoops and Movement Lesson

Children love hula hoops. They are inexpensive and can be used indoors. They can be easily manipulated by the child and make good targets or bases. Let the child's imagination make up games.

## PURPOSE

1. Improve agility and coordination
2. Learn to play with hoops.

## PREPARATION

One hoop per child

## PARTICIPATION

1. Use the hoop like a jump rope.
2. Walk while rolling the hoop like a tire.
3. Toss and catch the hoop.
4. Walk through the hoop as it is rolling.
5. Circle the hoop using an arm.

6. Circle the hoop around your waist. Keep going for as long as possible!
7. Toss the hoop to a partner without letting it touch the ground.
8. Spin the hoop and run around it as many times as possible before the hoop falls.
9. Roll the hoop at a target.
10. Toss the hoop around an object.

## BALL SKILLS UNIT

Ball handling builds perceptual skills. These skills are involved in anticipating an object's speed, direction, and timing. In sports, it means how to avoid being hit by a ball or hitting the ball with a bat successfully (timing.) Manipulating objects develops hand/eye and foot/eye coordination, fine motor and gross motor skills. Early competency in handling objects provides a firm foundation for more specialized sports skills that come later. Throwing, catching, and striking skills involve timing and coordination of many body parts. A good foundation for these skills should be laid in grades K through 3. Not only should the child experience these skills, but also gain knowledge in the principles behind efficient movement and manipulation skills. The following lesson plans are intended for grades K through 3. The activities are listed in a progressive order from simple activities to more complex activities (example: a simple skill of bouncing a ball with two hands must be learned before a more complex skill such as bouncing a basketball with one hand can be attempted.) An easy way to start is to to give a balloon to a pre-schooler and let them experiment.

## Ball Handling Lesson
### PURPOSE

1. Increase hand/eye and foot/eye coordination.
2. Improve the skills of dribbling, throwing, catching the ball.

### PREPARATION

A balloon for each pre-schooler, a Nerf ball for K–1 and an 8-inch playground ball for older children.

### PARTICIPATION
**Basic Perception**

1. Move the ball around a body part—waist, head, knee.
2. Sit on the ball and bounce on it.
3. Place the feet on the sides of the ball and jump up. Try to throw the ball up to the hands with your feet.
4. With a partner, stand back to back. Move the ball around the waists, necks, and knees.
5. Move the ball between the legs and over the head.
6. With a partner, sit on the floor 5 feet apart. Roll the ball back and forth, first with the left hand, then with the right hand, and finally, with both hands.
7. With a partner, bounce the ball back and forth.
8. Place the ball on the ground and jump over it; jump forward and backward.

**Catching**

In the primary grades, there are two main types of catches: the two-hand underhand catch and the two-hand overhand catch. The fundamentals to both are:

1. Keep the eyes on the ball until it is caught.
2. The arms should go out to meet the ball, then recoil back toward the body after contact to minimize the bouncing of the ball off the hands.
3. Hold the ball with the thumbs and fingers, not the palms.

## Throwing

1. Throw, roll, or shoot the ball at a target.
2. Throw the ball up, turn around, and catch it.
3. Throw the ball very high and catch it. (outdoors)
4. Throw the ball very high and clap the hands as many times as possible before it bounces. (outdoors)
5. Throw the ball very high and catch it on the first bounce. (outdoors)
6. Throw the ball high, turn around, and catch it on the first bounce.

## OVERHAND THROW

7. Do the above activities with different types of balls.
8. Throw the ball to a partner between the legs, like a football hike.
9. Throw the ball against a wall and catch it after one bounce.
10. Throw the ball at targets.
11. Throw the ball on the garage roof and catch it.
12 Throw the ball into a mini trampoline set against a tree.
13. Do the Overhand Throwing Lab (chapter)

## UNDERHAND SOFTBALL PITCH
### Dribble

1. Kneel on the right knee and bounce the ball with the right hand. All fingers should be touching the ball. Dribble the ball around the body.
2. Kneel on the left knee and bounce the ball with the left hand.
3. Stand, dribble the ball, keeping it waist high.

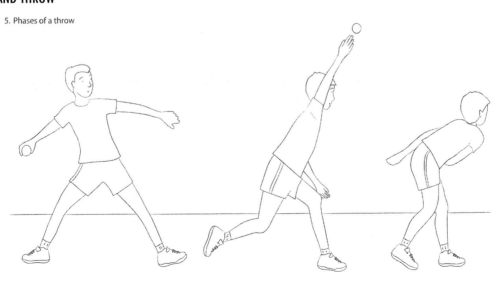

5. Phases of a throw

4. Dribble using left hand only, then right hand, then both hands.

5. Dribble the ball as close to the ground as possible; then, as high as possible.

6. Move while dribbling the ball.

7. Dribble the ball while not looking at the ball.

8. Dribble the ball with the eyes closed.

9. Dribble the ball around an obstacle course.

10. Do the Basketball Dribbling Lab (chapter 7)

### Bounce

1. Bounce the ball to a partner.

2. Have the ball bounce to partner's waist.

3. Bounce the ball to a partner using only the right hand, then the left hand, and finally, both hands.

4. Bounce the ball against a wall and catch it.

5. Bounce the ball toward a target on the wall.

6. Bounce the ball successively in hopscotch squares.

7. Bounce the ball while running

8. Bounce the ball, turn around, and catch it after one bounce.

### Striking and Kicking a Ball

There are two types of striking skills; one is striking with an implement (bat or racquet,) and the second is striking with the hand or foot (soccer, volleyball.) The common fundamentals are:

A. Keep the eye on the ball until it has been hit.

B. Follow-through with the swinging motion after the hit.

C. Maintain a firm grip on the implement. Do not throw it.

1. Strike the ball up with your hand and catch it after one bounce.

2. Strike the ball with your hand for distance.

3. Strike the ball into a wall and catch it after one bounce.

4. Strike the ball so it hits a target.

5. Play croquet outdoors, indoors with a tennis ball.

6. Kick a ball for distance. Do the Lab Soccer Kick (chapter 7.)

7. Kick a stationary ball into a box lying on its side or through the legs of a chair.

8. Kick a stationary ball to a partner.

9. Kick a rolling ball to a partner.

10. Kick a ball into a wall and stop the rebound with your feet.

11. Trap the ball by letting it roll under your foot with the toes pointed up.

12. Kick and trap a ball using your non dominant leg.

13. Kick the ball at a target.

14. Do the Lab Soccer Foot Trap (chapter 7.)

15. Play Four Square (chapter 4.)

16. Play Kids Handball (chapter 4.)

17. Play Balloon Volleyball (chapter 4.)

In striking with an implement (bat or racquet,) it is important to "snap the wrist" just as the ball contacts the bat. This motion will add more force to your swing. A drill to teach the timing of the "snap" is to "fling" the bat into a backstop using the wrist. Face a fence or backstop and swing a bat at an imaginary ball. At the moment the ball meets the bat, snap the wrists to move the bat faster. After the wrists have been snapped, release the bat. The student will be able to see that as he snaps the wrist faster, the bat will fly farther.

Practice striking by playing sock-it. Place a ball (tennis ball, softball) in a sock. Tie a rope to the sock and hang it from a tree branch or garage rafter. Practice striking stance and swing (tennis, baseball, racquetball) without having to chase the ball or break windows.

## Paddle Ball Lesson
### PURPOSE
Improve striking ability with hand extension (tennis, baseball).

### PREPARATION
One tennis ball or Nerf ball and one paddle or racquetball racquet per child.

### PARTICIPATION
1. Bounce the ball on the floor using the paddle.
2. Hit the ball into the air using the paddle.
3. Run and bounce the ball with the paddle.
4. Hit the ball into a wall and hit the rebound.
5. Ask your child: How many times can you keep hitting it before you miss? Keep count.
6. Hit the ball for distance with the paddle.
7. Bounce the ball once and hit it at a target.
8. Play Four Square using paddles.
9. Play Kids' Handball.

## Soccer Lead-up Activities Lesson
### PURPOSE
- Improve control in kicking, rolling, stopping a ball.
- Learn the rules of soccer.

### PREPARATION
One ball per child. Six milk cartons (for goals and bases).

### PARTICIPATION
1. Kick the ball to a partner using the inside of the foot.
2. Kick into a wall and stop the rebound using foot trap.
3. The partner stops the ball with a foot trap, placing the foot on top of the ball.
4. Kick at targets.
5. Play Home Run Kickball
6. Practice shooting at the goal with a goalie.
7. Play Keep Away using only the feet.
8. Do the soccer labs.
9. Play Speedy Soccer.

## Basketball Lead-up Activities Lesson
### PURPOSE
Improve skills of basketball, catching, throwing, shooting, dribbling.

### PREPARATION
1. One ball per child. (Basketball or Nerf ball, 8-inch utility ball, rolled up socks.)
2. Basketball hoop or trash can.

### PARTICIPATION
1. Dribble right hand, left hand, alternating hands.
2. Two-hand chest pass.
3. Two-hand overhead pass.
4. Two-hand bounce pass.
5. Shooting from different locations and distances.
6. Play horse. Take turns shooting. If you make a basket, the next shooter must make a basket from the same spot. If he misses the shot, he gets a letter. The first

player to miss five shots (or spell horse) loses.

7. Play Steal. While dribbling a ball, try to bat the ball away from other players. Try to guard your ball.

8. Play No Dribble Basketball. No dribbling is allowed. Good for indoors.

9. How many baskets can you make in one minute?

10. Do the basketball labs (chapter 7).

11. Play Lightning Basketball (chapter7).

## JUGGLING UNIT

### Juggling is good for coordination

Find three balls. Something about the size and weight of a small apple is about right. You need something with the right weight so that you can really feel the weight when the object lands in your hand. Lacrosse balls are great and not too expensive and they come in different colors, which makes them more fun to watch. Tennis balls are too light; golf balls are too small; soft-balls are too big. The soft juggling balls they sell are good but expensive (the advantage to those is they don't roll away when you drop them.) However, lacrosse balls can work if you practice standing over a bed—that way, the balls won't roll away.

1. To start juggling, imagine two spots about a foot in front of your forehead: one to the right, one to the left, and about 8 inches apart. These are your focus points. Hold your arms at waist level with your hands naturally out in front of you. This is your *rest* position. Starting with a ball in your

**Ball Skill Inventory**

Can the student perform the following activities?

Name _____

| Yes | No | |
|-----|-----|-----|
| ❏ | ❏ | Throws the ball to a partner and catches the ball. |
| ❏ | ❏ | Throws the ball at a wall target and hits the target 5 out of 10 times. |
| ❏ | ❏ | Dribbles a ball with control. |
| ❏ | ❏ | Dribbles a ball with control while walking. |
| ❏ | ❏ | Dribbles a ball with control with eyes closed. |
| ❏ | ❏ | Strikes a ball up 3 times consecutively. |
| ❏ | ❏ | Kicks a ball and hits a target. |
| ❏ | ❏ | Shoots a ball into a basketball goal 5 out of 10 times. |
| ❏ | ❏ | Bounces a ball on the floor with a paddle 5 consecutive times. |
| ❏ | ❏ | With a paddle, hits the ball against a wall 5 consecutive times. |
| ❏ | ❏ | Stops a rolling ball with a one foot trap. |

right hand and your left hand empty, toss the ball across to the left imaginary spot and catch it in your left hand. Now toss it back from your left hand across to the imaginary spot on the right and catch it in your right hand.

Keep your focus on hitting the imaginary spots, and concentrate on not throwing too high, too low, too far out, or too close to yourself. You'll be surprised to find that, soon, you won't have to watch the ball to catch it! If you throw it reasonably well, your catching hand will know where the ball is without you looking, and you will have no trouble catching it. Here is an important tip: don't worry about catching; instead, worry about tossing well.

2. Now, add another ball. Two balls will be easy: just throw the second ball up as the first ball starts to reach its peak (the highest point before descending.) Don't worry if the balls occasionally collide.

3. Once you have the pattern down for two balls, add a third ball. Throw the third ball when the second ball is at its peak height. At this point, the first ball should be passing from one hand to another. Don't worry about catching it at first. Just get used to throwing all three balls at the right times.

Anyone can do it if they practice, practice—and practice some more!

## TUMBLING AND GYMNASTICS UNIT

Stunts and tumbling are a pillar in physical education because they encourage a student to develop in the basic areas of balance, coordination, flexibility, agility, endurance, and strength.

Stunts and tumbling can be done with little to no equipment. However, students wanting to pursue more advanced gymnastics will need more equipment than can be supplied at home, in which case you should enroll them in a class.

I have not included all the stunts or all the teaching instructions for stunts and tumbling because this would be a separate book by itself. Rather, my intent is to list the activities that can be done at home. Note that, below, the appropriate grade range at which a child has the physical capabilities of doing an activity is listed in brackets.

Numerous books on gymnastics are available at your local library to supplement your needs in gymnastics. I feel one of the best teaching manuals is *A Manual For Tumbling and Apparatus Stunts*, by Ryser and Brown.

## Basic Elementary Stunts and Tumbling Lesson
### PURPOSE
1. Builds shoulder and arm strength.
2. Builds coordination.
3. Introduction to more advanced gymnastics.

### PREPARATION
For padding, use the grass, carpeted room, a number of scattered rugs, or a mat.

### STUNTS
1. Dog Walk—Walk on the hands and feet with the stomach off the floor. (K–2)
2. Duck Walk—Squat down, place hands behind the back to form a tail, and walk around. (K–2)

3. Inchworm—Bend down and place the hands on the floor. Keep the feet stationary and walk on the hands, away from the feet. Then, keep the hands stationary and walk on the feet toward the hands. In this way, the body will slowly move forward, like an inchworm.

5. Frog Hop—Short hops from a squatting position.

6. Log Roll—Lay on the stomach with arms extended straight over the head. Roll around. (K–2)

7. Tightrope Walk—Walk down a line on the floor. (K–2)

8. Side Roll—Put knees to the chin. Roll into a ball. Roll around the room. (K–2)

9. Crab Walk—Sit on the floor with knees bent, lean back on the arms with bottom off the floor. Walk on the feet and hands, first forward, then backwards, and then sideways. (K–3)

10. Mule Kick—Stand, then lean forward and put body weight onto hands; kick feet back and upward. Land on your feet again. (K–3)

11. One Foot Stand—Stand on one foot. (K–3)

12. Rocker—Sit on the floor. Bring knees to chest and rock on the back. (K–3)

13. Seal Walk—Lay on the stomach. From a push-up position, move forward using the arms. The legs are immobile and the feet will be dragged along the floor. (K–3)

14. Pretzel Stand-up—Sit cross-legged on the floor with the arms folded across the chest. Then, stand up without uncrossing the feet or unfolding the arms. It's tricky!

15. Knee Dip—Stand on the right foot. Bend the left leg back and grab the ankle. Gradually bend the right knee until the left knee touches the floor. Return to the starting position. (K–up)

16. Seal Slap—Begin by lying on the stomach with hands under the shoulders. Push off with the hands. Clap hands while in mid-air and return to starting position. (3–6)

17. Arabesque—Stand on the right leg and raise the left leg to a position parallel to the floor. Bend forward at the waist so the trunk is parallel with the floor.

18. Upswing—Begin in a kneeling position. Vigorously swing your arms forward and upward and stand up without moving the feet. (2–6)

19. Snap-up—Start lying down on the back. In one rapid movement, bend the knees towards the head, vigorously extend the legs upward and forward, and land on your feet in a squatting position. (4–up)

## STANDS

1. Knee Stand—An introduction to the headstand. Place the hands and head on the floor. Slowly bring the right knee to the right elbow and rest it on the elbow. Do the same with the left knee.

2. Head Stand—Form a triangle with the hands and forehead. Put the knees on the elbows and balance there. Slowly raise the legs upward until the body forms a straight line. Keep the back straight. Keep the weight on the forehead and not the top of the head. (1–6)

3. Hand Stand—Begin with the hands shoulder width apart on the mat. Kick the right foot upward, followed by the left foot.

Stand on the hands. Eyes should be looking at the mat. (4–6)

4. Forearm Balance—Do a modified hand stand, with the forearms on the mat. (6–up)

5. Shoulder Stand—Begin on the back, then lift the feet above the head and use the hands to help lift the hips off the floor.

## ROLLS

1. Forward Roll—Begin in a squat position. Push forward from the toes and tuck the chin to the chest. Roll forward and land with weight on the hands. Continue to roll onto the shoulders. Push off with the hands and return to a squat position. Have beginners start squatting on a low bench or large phone book. (K–3)

2. Backward Roll—Begin in a squat position. Push off with the hands and roll backward. Keep the chin tucked to the chest. When the weight is on the shoulders, push off with the hands and return to the starting position. (1–3)

3. Dive Roll—Dive over an object and land on your hands. Continue the motion of a forward roll. (3–6)

4. Cartwheel—Face the mat with the right foot forward and the arms raised upward. Bend backward slightly and shift the weight to the left foot. Then whip the arms forward and down, bending forward at the waist, and shifting the weight to the right foot while raising the left foot. Place the right hand in front of the right foot. As the hand strikes the mat, push off with the right foot. Place the left hand in front of the right hand. Both feet should be straight up with the hips and knees straight. As the body continues in motion, lift the right hand as the left foot touches the mat in front of the left hand. The right foot then lands in front of the left foot and you end standing in an upright position. Doing this along a wall will help the child place the feet and hand in a straight line. (3–6)

5. Round Off—A modified cartwheel where both feet land together and the body faces the direction the run was from. (3–up)

6. Headspring—This is an introduction to the handspring. From a short run, place hands and head on mat or chair. Jump up into a head stand. Let the body fall forward and arch the back. Push with the hands. This will force the upper body up.

7. Handspring—From a short run go into a hand stand, continue to bring the feet up and over. Land with both feet on the ground. (4–up)

## COMBINATIONS OF STUNTS AND TUMBLING

1. Do five or six stunts of your choice in a row for a routine.

2. Backward roll into a headstand.

The walkover (4–up), back flip (6–up), and front flip (6–up) are stunts that are dangerous to teach unless you know how to "spot" properly. I recommend you read in a good gymnastics manual how to "spot" and teach these stunts.

## BALANCE BEAM

Many of the previous stunts can be done on a balance beam. Place a wood 2x4 or 4x4 (8 to 12 feet long) on the floor for an instant "beam."

Make an incline beam by placing a brick under one end. Encourage the child to look straight ahead and focus his eyes on an object. This will increase their balancing skill. Scatter objects (beanbags, peanuts) along the beam for him to jump over and pickup.

Stunts: V-sit, front scale, skip across, hop across, walk forward and backward, squat and half-turn. (1–6)

### RINGS — USE THE RINGS ON A SWING SET

1. Skin the Cat—From a straight arm hang, bring the legs and hips over the head and continue to rotate until the legs extend downward. Your child may drop to their feet or reverse the movement. (1–6)
2. Bird Nest Hang—From a hang, raise the feet overhead and hook the toes in the rings.
3. Inverted Straight Hang—From a hang, bring the legs and hips over the head. Slowly raise the legs to an upright position. (2–6)
4. Straight Arm Support—Lift your child up from a standing position to a position where his or her weight is on your palms and your arms are straight down, with the hips higher than the rings.

### PARTNER ACTIVITIES

1. Leap Frog—One partner squats. The back partner rests his hands on his partner's shoulders and leaps over with his legs spread. (K–3)
2. Wheelbarrow—One partner lays on the floor. The other partner grabs his ankles. The front partner then walks on his hands with the other partner walking behind. (1–6)

3. Handspring Over Partner—Do a handspring over a kneeling partner. (4–up)

## SWIMMING UNIT

One of the most important safety and recreational skills a child should learn is swimming. The number of swimming facilities, public and private, have increased through the years. Access is available through YMCAs, schools, apartment complexes, health clubs, and public beaches. YMCAs and city recreation departments typically offer good lessons for a modest fee. I have not included all the swimming skills or the complete teaching instructions for swimming because this would be a separate book by itself. My intent is to list swimming activities I believe home educators can introduce and to give them a short lesson plan to introduce each skill. Numerous books on swimming can be found in the library or purchased from the Red Cross to supplement your swimming instruction. Children love to swim, and it is excellent for fitness training. Each time you visit the pool, devote 10 minutes to developing your child's swimming skills by using one of the following lesson plans. The activities are listed in the approximate order of beginner to more advanced skills.

## Blowing Bubbles

The purpose of this drill is to help your child overcome fear of placing his or her face in the water. You should be in the water with your child.

1. Demonstrate by placing your face in the water and blow out, making large bubbles.
2. Have the child imitate you.

3. Have a game of who can make the loudest noise blowing bubbles.

4. Who can make the noise for the longest time?

## Bobbing

The purpose is to help a beginner in rhythmic breathing. You should be in the water with your child.

1. Hold on to the side of the pool and bob up and down holding your breath.

2. Try to maintain a rhythm of breaking the surface every 2 seconds.

3. After the student has mastered this, take a breath, submerge, and blow air out for 5 seconds and surface.

4. Repeat the cycle several times.

5. Repeat the exercise varying the length of time you take to exhale.

## Rhythmic Breathing Drill

The purpose is to imitate the front crawl breathing.

1. Stand in waist-deep water.

2. Extend the right arm and hold the side of the pool.

3. Take a breath and place the face in the water so the water is at the hairline.

4. Exhale, blowing bubbles.

5. Turn the face to the side, away from the extended arm. Keep the head in the water.

6. Inhale through the mouth, then turn the face back into the water.

## Flutter Kick

1. Hold the side of the pool.

2. Kick the legs from the hip.

3. Try not to bend the knees too much.

4. The heels will touch the water surface.

5. Repeat this drill with a kick board. Flutter kick across the pool.

6. Try to flutter kick across the pool without a board and with the face in the water.

## Swimming Underwater

The purpose of this drill is to help relieve the fear of swimming underwater. You should be in the water with your child.

1. Have the child stand with his back to the pool wall.

2. Duck under the water and push off from the side of the pool with the feet.

3. The child will swim through the adult's legs.

4. Repeat the drill away from the side of the pool.

## Front Float

1. Stand in chest-deep water.

2. Extend arms over head.

3. Bend over until arms and chest are in the water.

4. Push off with the feet.

5. Glide slowly forward.

## Jellyfish Float

1. Stand in chest-deep water.

2. Bend at the waist and grab the ankles.

3. The feet should rise off the bottom.

4. The head should be pointed down and the back slightly out of the water.

5. See how long the breath can be held.

## Back Float

1. Stand in chest-deep water.

2. Lean back until water is over the shoulders.

3. Look at the ceiling and lay the head back until the ears get wet.

4. Hold the breath.

5. Push off lightly with the feet. Push the chest up.

6. Prevent the feet from rising towards the surface.

7. Kick lightly with the feet to propel the body through the water.

## Elementary Back Stroke

9. Elementary backstroke

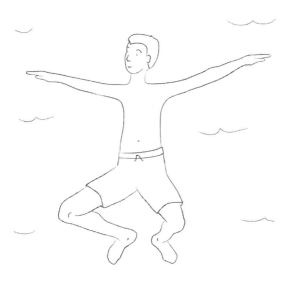

The first stroke for beginners is the elementary back stroke because the face stays out of the water, and it is not a tiring stroke. A beginner can travel great distances with this stroke.

1. Float on the back.

2. Both arms are drawn up to the armpits, with the elbows in. At the same time, the legs pull up and out with the knees together.

3. Then, in one fluid motion, the arms extend outwards and, keeping elbows straight, forcefully push down to the side of the

body again. At the same time, the legs are pushed down and together. This is the power phase.

5. Glide with the arms at the side.

## Front Crawl Stroke

The front crawl or freestyle is the fastest stroke. The arms pull and recover alternately and the legs do a continuous flutter kick. There is no glide phase in this stroke.

1. During the arm recovery phase, the arm should come out of the water.

2. Imagine a string pulling the elbow up, out of the water.

3. The hand will leave the water near the hip.

4. The fingertips should enter the water directly ahead of the shoulder with arm fully extended down.

5. Pull your hand and forearm back with the elbow slightly bent.

6. The face should turn toward the pulling arm and a breath taken at the completion of the power stroke.

7. The head is rolled to the side for breathing, but keep the side of the head in the water.

8. The kick should be kept just under the surface and no more than the heel should break the surface.

## Side Stroke

The side stroke is not a competitive stroke but is valuable for life-saving purposes. It is one of the least tiring strokes.

1. Start on your right side in the water.

**The sequence is as follows:**

3. Pull with the left arm, scissor kick the legs, push the right arm in front of head and glide.

4. During the glide, the top arm (left) is kept by the side.
5. The bottom arm (right) is extended straight forward.
6. The legs are together.
7. The sequence is repeated. The face is out of the water at all times, looking at the side.

## Tread Water

The skill of treading water should be mastered by all swimmers. It is essential for safety.

1. Slowly draw the hands and forearms back and forth across the top of the water in a sculling action, with palms down.
2. A scissor or whip kick is done slowly.
3. Use only enough force to keep the face out of the water.
4. Do *not* try to keep the shoulders out of the water.

## Feet-First Surface Dive

This dive is used in unknown or dark waters.

1. Start by treading water.
2. Thrust your body vertically out of the water with a strong scissor kick.
3. Extend your arm high over your head and sink as deep as you can.

## Pike Surface Dive

1. From a front glide position, tuck the chin and pull the arms to the hips.
2. The legs will be parallel with the surface and the trunk vertical.
3. Lift the legs out of the water into a vertical position. (The person is now upside down in the water.)

4. Extend the arms to a position over the head and descend.

## Deck Dive

1. Start by kneeling by the pool side.
2. The toes of one foot should be curled over the edge of the pool.
3. Extend the arms over the pool with hands together.
4. Tuck the chin to chest.
5. Roll off the edge of the pool and reach for the bottom of the pool.

## Standing Deck Dive

1. Start in a standing position with toes of both feet curled over the edge of the pool.
2. Bend over at the waist.
3. Extend the arms over the head.
4. Bend over at the waist until the fingertips almost touch the water.
5. Roll forward until the head breaks the surface of the water.
6. When the fingertips do touch the water, push off with the feet with a small jump.

## Games in the Water

Described in chapter 4 Water Volleyball, Marco Polo, Keep The Ball Away, 500 Ball Catch, Tag

## RHYTHM UNIT: JUMP ROPE AND DANCE

It would be difficult to name a sports skill that does not involve rhythm. We run, swim, and dribble a ball in a rhythm. Music and rope jumping are excellent tools to introduce rhythm to children. Jumping rope is inexpensive, one of

HOME SCHOOL FAMILY FITNESS

the best aerobic activities, and can be done indoors.

## Single Jump Rope Lesson

Jumping rope is often thought of as a children's activity. However, it is a great activity for people of all ages. It is an excellent way to build aerobic endurance, coordination, and strength. It can be a lot of fun for everyone if you add a variety of stunts while jumping.

### PURPOSE

1. Learn to jump rope.
2. Improve coordination and rhythm.
3. Improve aerobic endurance.

### PREPARATION

One jump rope per child. Rope should be shoulder height with the rope under the feet. There are several kinds and thickness of rope that can be used for rope jumping. Probably ⅜ inch sash cord is the best and available in hardware stores. Any rope up to ½ inch in thickness is acceptable. If the rope is too light in weight, it can be difficult to spin.

### PARTICIPATION

1. Lay a rope on the ground. Jump over the rope with two feet together, forward and backward to a constant beat.
2. Hop on one foot. Do it without looking at the feet.
3. Tie a beanbag to the end of a 10-foot rope. Swing it in a circle while the child jumps over the rope. Jump as slowly as you can, as fast as you can. Hop on right foot, left foot, both feet, alternate feet.
4. Have the child swing the rope from behind

and overhead to a stop in front of the feet. Next, have him or her jump over the rope. Continue this process, speeding it up each time.

### SINGLE ROPE JUMPING

♦ When jumping, keep the upper arms close to the body with the elbows almost touching the sides. Have the forearms out at right angles and turn the rope by making small circles with the hands and wrists.
♦ Land on the balls of your feet.
♦ Try jumping to music, as it can keep the body moving in a steady rhythm.

### PROGRESSION TO LEARN BASIC STUNTS:

1. Rope turning forward and two-foot hop.
2. Rope turning backward and two-foot hop.
3. Rope turning forward and hop on one foot.
4. Rope turning backward and hop on one foot.
5. Rope turning forward and hop on right, then hop on left foot.
6. Rope turning backward and hop on right, then hop on left foot.
7. Rope turning forward and run forward.
8. Rope turning backward and run backward.
9. Rope turning forward and double speed the rope. The rope must make two full turns while the performer's feet are off the ground.
10. Rope turning backward and double speed. The rope must make two full turns while the performer's feet are off the ground.

## ADDITIONAL STUNTS:

### Basic Two-Foot Hop

Jump on both feet. Keep feet, ankles, and knees together. Hop over the rope. It can be done forward or backward.

### Rocker Step

Jump with one foot ahead of the other.

### Jump Turn

While jumping do a quarter-turn until you have rotated all the way around.

### Side Swing and Jump

1. Twirl rope to the left side.
2. Jump over the rope.
3. Twirl rope to right side.
4. Jump over rope.

### Side Hop

Hop to the left 4 to 6 inches with feet together. Hop right 4 to 6 inches with feet together.

### Cross Arms

Cross arms and jump, return to basic hop.

### Double Under

Two rotations of the rope with one jump. This requires jumping higher than normal.

### Scissors Step

Jump with left foot ahead, jump and put right foot ahead.

## Long Rope Jumping

Long rope jumping may be performed with one or more students jumping over a rope turned by two people. The rope may be turned by one person if one end is tied to a stationary object (post, railing.) There are two ways to turn the rope. The front door turning may be easier for beginners.

**Front door:** The jumper waits until the rope is moving down and away from him before he runs into the rope.

**Back door:** The jumper waits until the rope is at the highest peak and is moving downward before he runs into the rope.

The following progressions can be done by entering either front door or back door.

1. Run under the rope.
2. Run in, jump once, and run out.
3. Run in, jump several times, and run out.
4. Run in, jump on one foot, run out.
5. Run in, jump on one foot several times, run out.
6. Run in, jump making 1/4, 1/2, 3/4 or full turns with each jump, run out.
7. Run in, jump on alternate feet, run out.
8. Run in, touch the floor with hands on every other jump, run out.
9. Run in, take a squat position (on all fours) and jump in this position, run out.

The word *rhythm* in Greek means "measured motion or a cadence." Rhythmic motions are all around us. The waves beat the shore in rhythm. In the human body, the heart beats in rhythm. In sports, we may say that a shortstop fielded a ball and threw to first base with "perfect rhythm."

Rhythm is a foundational skill that can be mastered through dance. That is why I recommend 10% of the year's activities be devoted to dance for elementary children. For grades K through 1, you may consider 20% of the year devoted to rhythm and dance because if a gym is not available, dance can be done in a classroom and needs no equipment. Young children (K–1) often have trouble understanding the rules of games. The singing/dance games need little explanation and make class room management easier for the teacher.

Common singing games/dances done by elementary children are listed below. These dances teach basic rhythm and provide beginning steps for more advanced dances. A group of children are needed to do many dances, although the basic steps can be taught to one single child. Numerous tapes, records, and videos are available from libraries. Teaching instructions usually come with the tapes.

## SINGING GAMES FOR PRIMARY GRADES

| | | |
|---|---|---|
| Baa, Baa Black Sheep | circle | K |
| Hickory, Dickory, Dock | circle | K |
| Ring Around the Rosy | circle | K–1 |
| Farmer in the Dell | circle | K–1 |
| The Muffin Man | circle | K–1 |
| London Bridge | line | K–1 |
| A Hunting We Will Go | line | 1–2 |
| Shoo Fly | circle | 2–3 |

### Baa, Baa Black Sheep (K)

| Measure | Song |
|---|---|
| 1–8 | Baa Baa black sheep, |
| | Have you any wool? |
| | Yes sir, yes sir, |
| | Three bags full. |
| 1–8 | One for my master, |
| | One for my dame, |
| | And one for the little boy |
| | Who lives in the lane. |

Single circle, facing center and hands joined. One child in center of circle

Eight walking steps right. Place hands on hips and nod on word "yes," hold three fingers up on word "three," and arms out to show a large bag.

Turn right and bow or curtsy.
Turn left and bow or curtsy.
Face center and bow or curtsy

### Hickory, Dickory, Dock (K)

| Measure | Song |
|---|---|
| 1–4 | Hickory, Dickory, Dock! |
| 5–8 | The mouse ran up the clock |
| 1–4 | The clock struck one, the mouse ran down, |
| 5–8 | Hickory, Dickory, Dock. |

Double circle with inside hands on partner's shoulder and both facing counterclockwise. One child is the "mouse," and the other the "clock."

Sway toward center of circle.

Sway toward outside. Stamp one foot, then the other.

Mouse runs clockwise around his partner then stamps feet as above. Clock claps hands on the word "one." Mouse runs counterclockwise. Repeat.

### Ring Around The Rosy (K–1)

Ring a round the rosy
A pocket full of posies,
Ashes, ashes
They all fall down.

Single circle, players join hands and face center. With hands joined, walk or skip around the circle. Drop to a squatting position.

# Farmer In The Dell (K–1)

| Measure | Song |
| --- | --- |
| 1–2 | The farmer in the dell, |
| 3–4 | The farmer in the dell, |
| 5–6 | Heigh-ho! the cherry-o, |
| 7–8 | The farmer in the dell. |
| 1–2 | The farmer takes a wife, |
| 3–4 | The farmer takes a wife, |
| 5–6 | Heigh-ho the cherry-o, |
| 7–8 | The farmer takes a wife. |
| 1–8 | The wife takes the child, etc. |
| 1–8 | The child takes the nurse, etc. |
| 1–8 | The nurse takes the dog, etc. |
| 1–8 | The dog takes the cat, etc |
| 1–8 | The cat takes the rat, etc. |
| 1–8 | The rat takes the cheese, etc., |
| 1–8 | The cheese stands alone |
| 1–8 | The farmer runs away, etc. |
| 1–8 | Repeat for each player as he leaves the center of the circle |

Single circle facing center with hands joined. One child (the farmer) is in the center of the circle. All walk left around circle singing the verse while the farmer looks for a wife. Continue to walk around the circle as the farmer chooses a wife who joins him at the center of the circle.

Repeat with the wife choosing a child.

Repeat, choosing a person for each verse.

Children in center crowd around cheese and clap their hands over the cheese's head, while circle players stand still, clap hands, and sing.

Continue walking as the farmer, then wife, etc., leave the center of the circle.

Cheese remains and becomes the new farmer.

# The Muffin Man (K–1)

| Measure | Song |
| --- | --- |
| 1–2 | Oh, have you seen the muffin man, |
| 3–4 | The muffin man, the muffin man, |
| 5–6 | Oh, have you seen the muffin man, |
| 7–8 | Who lives on Drury Lane. |
| 1–2 | Oh yes, we've seen the muffin man, |
| 3–4 | The muffin man, the muffin man |
| 5–6 | Oh yes, we've seen the muffin man, |
| 7–8 | Who lives on Drury Lane. |

Single circle facing center with one child (the "muffin man") in the center of the circle. Children join hands and circle to the left (walking or slowly skipping.)

Children in circle stand facing center and clap hands while singing "The Muffin Man." The child in center chooses a partner from the circle and brings them back to the center. This child becomes the new muffin man while the old muffin man returns to the circle.

# London Bridge (K–1)

London Bridge is falling down,
falling down, falling down.
London Bridge is falling down,
My fair lady.
Build it up with bricks and stones,
bricks and stones, bricks and stones.
Build it up with bricks and stones,
My fair lady.

Two children hold their arms up to form a bridge. Other children walk under the bridge. When the word lady is sung, the two students drop their arms around a person. The person the bridge falls on then becomes a new bridge person.

## A-Hunting We Will Go (1–2)

(Simplified version of Virginia Reel)

| Measure | Song |
| --- | --- |
| 1–4 | Oh, a-hunting we will go, a-hunting we will go, |
| 5–8 | We'll catch a fox and put him in a box. And then we'll let him go. |
| *Chorus* | |
| 1–8 | Tra, la, la, la, la, la, la |
| | Tra, la, la, la, la, la |
| | Tra, la, la, la, la, la |
| | La, la, la, la |
| | Tra, la, la, la, la, la |

## Shoo Fly (2–3)

| Measure | Song |
| --- | --- |
| 1–2 | Shoo, fly, don't bother me; shoo, fly, don't bother me. |
| 3–4 | Shoo, fly, don't bother me, For I belong to somebody. |
| 5–8 | Repeat 1-4 |
| 9–16 | I feel, I feel |
| | I feel like a morning star; |
| | I feel, I feel, |
| | I feel like a morning star. |

Double circle.

Players join hands and walk four steps toward center, then four steps backward.

Repeat twice.

Partners join hands and walk around each other clockwise. On last "morning star," all players raise their hands. The outside circle walks forward one person and they now have a new partner.

## HISTORY OF AMERICAN FOLK AND CHILDREN'S DANCE

Our Protestant ancestors in the 1600s and 1700s wrestled with the idea of dance. They composed a large number of dances they felt were wholesome for their children to do in mixed gender groups. Today we call these songs American folk dances. Their list includes: "Virginia Reel," "Square Dance," "Skip to My Lou," "Buffalo Gals Won't You Come Out Tonight," "B.I.N.G.O.," "Pop Goes the Weasel," "Old Dan Tucker," and the square dances.

Dances with simple steps were called play-parties. Square dance is also a form of play-party dance.

## Dance Descriptions

### BAA, BAA BLACK SHEEP

♦ Single circle, facing center and hands joined. One child in center of circle.

♦ Eight walking steps right. Place hands on hips and nod on word "yes," hold three fingers up on word "three," and arms out to show a large bag.

♦ Turn right and bow or curtsy.

♦ Turn left and bow or curtsy.

♦ Face center and bow or curtsy.

### HICKORY, DICKORY, DOCK

♦ Double circle with inside hands on partner's shoulder and both facing counter-clockwise. One child is the "mouse," and the other the "clock."

♦ Sway toward center of circle.

♦ Sway toward outside. Stamp one foot, then the other.

♦ Mouse runs clockwise around his partner

then stamps feet as above. Clock claps hands on the word "one." Mouse runs counterclockwise. Repeat.

## FARMER IN THE DELL

- Single circle facing center with hands joined. One child (the farmer) is in the center of the circle.
- All walk left around circle singing the verse while the farmer looks for a wife.
- Continue to walk around the circle as the farmer chooses a wife who joins him at the center of the circle.
- Repeat with the wife choosing a child.
- Repeat, choosing a person for each verse.
- Children in center crowd around cheese and clap their hands over the cheese's head, while circle players stand still, clap hands, and sing.

## RING AROUND THE ROSY

- Single circle, players join hands and face center.
- With hands joined, walk or skip around the circle.

## THE MUFFIN MAN

- Single circle facing center with one child (the "muffin man") in the center of the circle. Children join hands and circle to the left (walking or slowly skipping.)
- Children in circle stand facing center and clap hands while singing "The Muffin Man." The child in center chooses a partner from the circle and brings them back to the center. This child becomes the new muffin man while the old muffin man returns to the circle.

## SHOO FLY

- Double circle.
- Players join hands and walk four steps toward center, then four steps backward.
- Repeat twice.
- Partners join hands and walk around each other clockwise. On last "morning star," all players raise their hands. The outside circle walks forward one person and they now have a new partner.

## A-HUNTING WE WILL GO

- Two parallel lines facing each other.
- Head couple joins inside hands and skip down between lines to the foot of the set.
- Head couple turns around, changes hands and skips back to head of set.
- All other players clap hands while head couple is skipping down and back.
- Head couple skips around the left side of the set followed by other couples. When the head couple reaches the foot of the line, they form an arch under which all other couples pass through. Head couple remains at the foot and the second couple becomes the new head couple.

## LONDON BRIDGE

- Two children hold their arms up to form a bridge. Other children walk under the bridge. When the word lady is sung, the two students drop their arms around a person. The person the bridge falls on then becomes a new bridge person.

## TRADITIONAL DANCES

| | | |
|---|---|---|
| Children's Polka | circle | 1–3 |
| Virginia Reel | line | 2–up |
| Mayim, Mayim | circle | 2–up |
| Tinikling | line | 2–up |
| Oh, Susanna | circle | 3–5 |
| O Johnny | circle | 4–up |
| Texas Star Square Dance | square | 5–up |

### TINIKLING (2–UP)

Philippine national dance commonly done in elementary schools.

**Purpose:** Develop rhythm and aerobics.

**Equipment:** One pair of 1½- or 2-inch PVC pipe 10 feet long and two 2x4s 3 feet long. Music in 4/4 time. Tinikling tape from the library.

**History:** This is the Philippine national dance. The dance imitates the movement of the tikling birds as they walk between grass stems or run over tree branches. Dancers imitate the tikling bird's legendary grace and speed by skillfully maneuvering between large bamboo poles. Tinikling means "bamboo dance" in English.

**Activity:** Six children at each station. Two children beat the sticks as the other children dance in and out of the poles (poles can be pvc pipe or electrical conduit). The beat pattern is two hits of poles on the 2x4s and then one hit of the poles together. First have the children do the steps with the poles stationary and no music. Next add the music. Next add music and moving poles. Tinikling is very similar to jump rope, but instead of a spinning rope, two bamboo poles are used. Visit this link to see a video of the dance: www.likha.org/galleries/tinikling.html.

**Basic Steps**

♦ **Singles:** When the poles are on the dancers right side (right foot lead) the foot work of two singles steps would be as follows:
- Count 1—Step on right foot between poles.
- Count 2—Step on left foot between poles.
- Count 3—Hop right foot outside poles
- Count 1—Step on left foot between poles.
- Count 2—Step on right foot between poles.
- Count 3—Step on left foot outside poles.
- Repeat.

♦ **Doubles:** The foot work for two doubles steps (with right side next to poles) would be:
- Count 1—Hop on both feet between poles.
- Count 2—Hop again on both feet between poles.
- Count 3—Hop on both feet outside (straddling) poles.
- Repeat.
- *Variation*—Turn 180 degrees on second hop inside of poles.

## Glossary of Dance Terms

These steps (calls) are basic to all traditional square, contra, and circle dances. Music was in 2/4 or 6/8 time. The old reels and jigs, such as "Turkey in the Straw," "Cripple Creek," "Pop Goes the Weasel," or "Arkansas Traveller" played by piano and/or fiddler, provided the music and beat.

**Head couple:** The couple nearest the music.

**Home:** The original starting position.

**Honor**: Ladies curtsy and gents bow.

**Bow:** The bow is done by the boys and is a bending forward of the trunk at the waist.

**Curtsy:** Done by the girls and is a deep knee bend.

**Corner:** When facing the center, the boy's corner is the girl on his left.

**Balance**: Join hands, bow and curtsy, then swing right forward while leaning back balancing on left, then reverse feet. (8 beats)

**Circle**: (8 hands around) All join hands and walk to left or right as instructed. Usually 8 steps then reverse for 8 more. (16 beats)

**Swing:** A couple swings once clockwise using one hand, two hands, or elbows. (8 beats of music)

**Promenade**: Facing to right, with lady on right, in skater's position, walk counter clockwise to home position. (usually 16 beats)

**Forward and Back**: Walk up to each other (almost touching) and backward to start. (8 beats)

**Do-Si-Do**: Walk forward, passing right shoulders around each other back to back, then walking backwards to start position. (8 beats)

**Sashay**: Joining hands and taking sliding steps to the side either face to face or facing same way (lady in front).

**Allemande Left:** Form a circle or square formation, all dancers face the center. The boy joins his left hand with the girl on his left ("Corner") and walks once around counterclockwise and back to starting position. (8 beats)

**Allemande Right:** Same as Allemande Left only in opposite direction.

**Promenade:** Partners join their inside hands and walk counterclockwise around the circle.

**Grand Right and Left**: Following an Allemande Left, each proceeds (gents counter clockwise, ladies clockwise) around the circle, weaving in and out, alternating using right and left hands (ladies with gents/ gents with ladies) 'til they meet their partners or reach home.

**Ladies Chain**: Ladies walk forward joining right hands as they pass, then joining left hands to gent opposite, who turns them around counter clockwise to stand on his right. Then "chain" back the same way to partner. (16 beats) (Sometimes done as a half)

**Right and Left Through**: Two couples walk forward, hands at sides and pass through each other (gents to the outside), then gents turn partners around to their right. (16 beats)

**Right or Left and Star**: Gents or ladies to center, grasping wrist of person to left, then walking together around. (8 beats then reverse 8 beats)

**Arch:** Two dancers join hands and raise arms upward to form an arch.

**Star or Wheel:** Two or more dancers join right hands in the center and walk forward or backward.

## Definitions of Formations:

**In the Quadrille or Square:** four couples arranged on four sides of a Square—Gents with Partners to right

**Corner Lady**: lady to your left

**Right-hand Lady**: lady of couple to your right

**Opposite Lady**: lady of couple across from you.

Your **Partner** can and will be called all sorts of names, but never a "lady" (to avoid confusion with the above three ladies).

The **Head Couple** (1) has their backs to the front of the hall.

**Head Couples**: the above (1) and the couple opposite them (3).

**Side Couples**: the couple to the right (2) and the couple to the left (4).

In a dance, the head couple usually goes through a series of figures with each of the couples around the square, then the couple to the right follows the same patterns until all four couples have gone through the series. Some dances use all the couples as head couples, like the Texas Star.

A fun note: Long ago, the square was the perfect dance for the limited space in frontier parlors and barns.

## In New England Contra Dancing and the Reels:
### (LINES OF 6–8 COUPLES — USUALLY "LADIES" FACE "GENTS")

**"Active" couples** (usually designated) dance and **"cast"** (pivot around the person to their right), thereby moving down the line. "Inactive" couples dance only when danced with, and move along the line on the left, toward the head. "Inactive" couples become "active" when they reach the head of the line.

A fun note: These "longways" dances were conducive to the long halls of New England architecture. These were often danced without calls, as instructions were not necessary once the figures had been taught. The dances were usually not as intricate as the squares.

## In Circle Dances:
### (AN EVEN NUMBER OF COUPLES ALTERNATE FACING FORWARD OR BACK AROUND THE CIRCLE)

Pairs of couples dance with each other through a series of steps. Then, they **"pass through"** the alternate couples, who are moving either counter-clockwise (through) or clockwise (around) to the next couples in the circle. They repeat the steps with the new couples, etc.

A fun note: These dances were originally done outdoors on warm nights in the South, where there was plenty of room for a circle.

# Rules and Teaching Labs for Sports

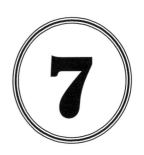

## PHYSICAL EDUCATION LABS

"A picture is worth a thousand words." Have you ever watched a mother feed her child? You have probably noticed how often she opens her mouth as she puts the spoon to her child's lips. This may look funny, but, in fact, the mother is modeling the action she wants the child to do, for her child to follow. People have done this for centuries because it works!

Similarly, physical skills can be learned by watching someone else do them correctly. Then, the skills are refined by repetitive practice: doing is learning.

The labs included in this book are designed to give the child a guided experience in physical activity. As the child performs an action, another person (parent or sibling) observes and records on the lab sheet what he sees. Better yet, the activity can be videotaped and the performer can observe him or herself, and record what improvements or changes can be made.

Each lab provides hints and instructions on how to perform the exercise correctly, and includes a list of what skills are used. Most of these labs can be done by children of any age; however, children ages 4 to 8 will need the help of an adult in the labs. Children ages 9 and up can do them on their own, but if they get feedback from others they will learn more. In the following labs, left-handers will need to change the right and left directions around.

Start with the walking & running correctly technique checklist, below. Then move on to sports. The following pages include the basic rules, skills, drills and labs for these common recreational sports.

Floor Hockey
Soccer
Football
Basketball

Softball
Volleyball
Tennis
Ultimate Frisbee

## Technique Checklist

The technique checklist is a tool to help the instructor give specific help in improving the sport skills. By observing one part of the student's body as he/she does the skill, the instructor can give detailed teaching tips. I have had students, fourth grade and up, teach each other sport skills from these sheets. I have the students pair up and the observer watch and record his observations. When the sheet is completed, the observer explains what he saw and gives suggestions for improvement. Students can be videotaped and the tape critiqued. This could be used as homework to be completed at home and returned the next class period.

# LAB: WALKING & RUNNING CORRECTLY TECHNIQUE CHECKLIST

Performer's Name _____

## PURPOSE

Learn to walk and run correctly.

Some people have developed a habit of walking with the toes pointed in or pointed out. Walking with the feet in these positions will add stress to the joints of the knee, ankle, and hip. Years of walking improperly can cause permanent damage to the joint. Normal foot placement for walking range from straight ahead to 10 degrees pointed out. During sprinting, toes should point straight ahead.

## Lab Activity (part I):

1. Wet the bottom of your bare feet.
2. Walk on a dry cement sidewalk or basement floor.
3. Observe the tracks you made.
4. Compare your tracks to the diagram at the right.
5. Are you walking correctly? If not, work at trying to make the correct tracks. You can overcome a bad habit by consciously walking correctly for a couple of weeks.

## Lab Activity (part II):

The purpose of this lab is to correct your jogging form. Running with proper form will prevent injuries to the ankle and knee. Jog slowly while someone observes you from the front, side, and back. The observer will look at one item from the checklist at a time and record a yes or no. Did you get "yes" for all the questions? If not, run again trying to correct your errors. Videotape the runner and have him use this checklist on himself.

### JOGGING CHECKLIST

| | | Yes | No |
|---|---|---|---|
| 1. | Toes are pointed straight ahead. | Yes | No |
| 2. | Knees are moving straight ahead. | Yes | No |
| 3. | Foot lands on the heel. | Yes | No |
| 4. | Elbows are bent at a 90-degree angle. | Yes | No |
| 5. | Palms are down and the wrist loose. | Yes | No |
| 6. | Erect body (not round-shouldered). | Yes | No |

Jogging is slow running with the heel touching the ground with each step. Sprinting is fast running with the heel never touching the ground. Sprinting is done on your toes.

7. While sprinting, do the feet hit the ground on the toes without the heels touching?                    Yes          No

# FLOOR HOCKEY

Rollerblading and street hockey are especially popular with kids these days. In fact, floor hockey is an excellent aerobic activity, as well as being a game. Its rules are similar to soccer, ice hockey, and street hockey. It is a moderately expensive sport and will cost approximately $100 to equip a class with 15 sticks. For instructional purposes any ball will work, but tennis balls are best.

## Basic Rules

The playing area should resemble a hockey rink and can be an entire gymnasium floor, parking lot, ice rink, tennis court, dead end street, or a grass lawn. Goals can be made of cardboard boxes, gymnastic mats, cones, or tape on a wall. Balls or pucks can be used. It can be played in Rollerblades or shoes.

The game begins with a face-off at midfield. The puck is dropped between two players. Each team attempts to advance the puck down field and to score a goal. Each team also tries to prevent the opponents from scoring. The goalkeeper is the only player allowed to handle the puck with his hands.

For the safety of the children the high sticking rule should be enforced. A high sticking penalty is given anytime a player has the head of his stick above his shoulder.

- Typically a team has five players plus a goalie.
- The game begins with face-off at centerline and resumes there after each goal.
- A face-off is called when ball is out of play, thrown, or caught by any player other than goalie. The official will drop ball during face-off.
- The ball may be stopped by hand, but not held, passed, or advanced by hand.
- Typically two 12-minute running time halves are played with no time-outs.
- A goal is scored when a player hits, sweeps, or pushes the ball into the net directly off stick or it is deflected off one of their teammates or a defensive player into the net.
- A player may advance the ball with their feet, but may not kick it directly into the net to score. If a player kicks the ball and it deflects off defensive player into net—the goal counts.
- A ball cannot be thrown into the goal to score.
- When a goalie catches or stops the ball, they must be given room to release it to one of their players by hand or stick. If a goalie falls onto a ball and is unable to release it, face-off is called to the front of the goal.

## Penalties

- HIGH STICKING: anytime the stick is raised above normal shoulder height.
- SLASHING: intentional or unintentional hitting with stick.
- INTERFERENCE AND CHARGING: anytime an opposing player pushes a player out of position.
- ELBOWING: using one's elbow to hit an opponent.
- CROSS CHECKING: use of stick to push opponent out of the way.
- TRIPPING AND HOOKING: use of stick to trip or hold back an opponent from playing the ball.

When a player commits a penalty, they are removed from the game for one minute.

## Variation:

Mega-Floor Hockey—A modification of the rules in an instructional setting to give more children an opportunity to handle the puck.

2 to 6 players per team. 3 to 6 teams.

Each team has one ball and one goal.

The goals are scattered around the perimeter of the playing area.

The first team to score a goal on each of the other teams wins.

## Basic Skills

The skills required for floor hockey are similar to soccer, and floor hockey should be considered a lead-up game to soccer. You should do your floor hockey unit before you teach the soccer unit.

The hands should be placed 12 to 18 inches apart on the stick. The spacing of the hands allows for better puck control and will help prevent high sticking. Most beginners will try to swing incorrectly by using a golf swing.

## DRILLS

**1. Steal Game** (K–up)

Equipment: approximately half as many balls as students

One stick for every student.

Skill: dribbling, defense

Students who have a ball must dribble it around the area using their stick. Students without a ball try to steal a ball. Stop every minute. Students with a ball are awarded one point. Use of the hands is not allowed.

**2. Shuttle Dribble Drill** (K–up)

Equipment: 4 balls, 4 to 6 sticks, 4 to 6 cones

Skill: dribbling

This is a relay race. Divide the students into four squads. Place the cones or chairs at mid-court. One player at a time must dribble the ball out to the cone using their stick, around the cone twice, and back to the next person in line. The next person does the same. Each team is awarded one point for each person who dribbles out and back. Have them do it continuously for 4 minutes. You will not need to have an equal number of students on each team if you use a time limit.

Variation: Have the student dribble out to the cone and then kick the ball back to the next person in line. After they kick the ball they return to the end of the line.

**3. Goal Shooting Drill** (K–up)

Equipment: 4 to 6 balls, mats, pails, or tape to mark goals approximately 6 to 8 feet wide, 4 to 6 sticks.

Skill: kicking accurately, goalie skills

Divide the students into squads of 3 to 6 students each. One student plays goalie while another student shoots the ball from 15 feet way. The goalie goes to the back of the squad line, the shooter becomes goalie, and the next student in line is the shooter.

**4. Goal Run Drill** (K–up)

Equipment: one ball for each student, two goals marked at opposite ends of the gym one stick for each player.

Skill: shooting accurately, dribbling, goalie skills

Two students play goalie. The rest of the students dribble and must shoot at

Goal A from a distance of 10 feet or greater. They keep trying until they score a goal on Goal A. They then dribble to Goal B and keep shooting until they make a goal. Then repeat. Have the students keep track of how many goals they make. Change goalies every 3 minutes until everyone has a chance.

Variation: Add one defensive back to each end to help the goalie defend the goal.

**5. Clean Your Backyard Drill** (K–4)

Equipment: tennis balls and stick for each player

Skill: passing

Students are divided into two groups. The midcourt basketball line divides the court into two areas. Team A must stay within its assigned half court and Team B in its assigned half court. The balls are tossed out and each group tries to pass balls out of their court into the other team's court. At the end of 2 minutes the whistle is blown and a count is taken of the number of balls on each court. The team with the fewest amount of balls gets one point. The hands may not be used. Repeat.

Variation: Each team tries to pass balls so they hit the back wall in the opponent's court. One point is awarded for each ball that touches the back wall. At the end of 5 minutes, start over.

**6. Sideline Floor Hockey Game** (K–up)

Equipment: 2 to 3 balls, 3 to 5 sticks per team

Regular basketball courts are the boundaries.

Skills: all soccer skills

Divide the students into two teams. Assign a number to each member of a team

(Mary is 1, Ted is 2, Mark is 3, Jill is 4 . . . ) until all students have a number. The students whose number you call (3,4,5) will run onto the playing area.

Example: The teacher calls numbers 1, 2, or 3. Three players from each team will run onto the court and play the game.

Those students whose numbers were not called must stand out-of-bounds along their assigned side line. If a ball goes out-of-bounds, those students standing out-of-bounds may play it and pass the ball to teammates. Rotate players every 3 to 4 minutes.

**Variation:** Use two or three balls at the same time. This will give the less skilled players more opportunity to handle the ball. The first ball to score ends the play and new numbers are called and fresh players come in. Three or four players per team at a time works best.

**7. Four Goal Floor Hockey** (3–up)

Equipment: 4 balls, 4 goals, sticks for all players

Skills: all soccer skills

Divide the class into four teams. The goals are placed in the four corners of the playing area. Four or more balls are put into play. Teams try to score on other goals. When a goal is scored, the goalie throws the ball back to midfield or to a teammate. The team with the fewest amount of goals scored on its goal wins.

**8. Hockey Rink Floor Hockey** (3–up)

Equipment: hockey rink with boards or tennis court, one ball

Skills: all soccer skills

Playing soccer outdoors in an ice rink allows the students to play and practice the skills more by spending less time chasing the ball. The less skilled players can play more easily.

# SOCCER

A game like soccer, kemari, was played around 600 B.C. in Japan. The Greeks also played a similar game called harpaston. This game was played by the Romans and eventually made its way to England, where our current rules developed. Soccer is played in more countries in the world than any other sport. Soccer is an excellent aerobic activity and is good for children because of the limited expense (a ball and two goals,) its potential for participation by many people, and its relatively simple rules.

## Basic Rules

Soccer skill instruction can start in first grade, and by fifth grade, the children should have learned a majority of the skills. Modified "lead-up" games should be used for instruction most of the time, because you can focus the students on a single skill and give equal practice time to all students by preventing the better players from monopolizing the play. The students can play the regular soccer rules outside of class.

What is soccer? Soccer is a game of running and kicking a ball with the feet. The use of the hands and arms is prohibited (with the exception of the goalkeeper). The game is played by two teams of eleven players who attempt to advance the ball toward the opponent's goal. A point is scored when the ball crosses the goal line between the goal posts and under the goal crossbar. The goal is 24 feet wide and 8 feet high.

The playing field is roughly the size of a football field. In collegiate play, the game is divided into two 45-minute halves with a 10 minute intermission.

### RULES FOR GOALKEEPER

The goalkeeper is a designated player and is usually given a different colored shirt so that the umpires and opponents can distinguish him from other players. While within the goal penalty box area, the goalkeeper has special privileges. He may: (1) catch, throw, punt, drop-kick, roll, or bounce the ball once; (2) not be interfered with by an opponent; and (3) walk not more than four steps before putting the ball into play. He loses all these privileges when he leaves the penalty box area.

### KICK-OFF

The game is started from the center circle of the field. The ball must be place-kicked into the opponents' half of the field. Before the ball is kicked, all players must be on their half of the field. Players of the other team cannot be within ten yards of the ball. The player who does the kick-off cannot play the ball again until another player touches it. Typically, the person kicking-off tries to kick the ball to a team mate.

### OUT-OF-BOUNDS RULES

Any player is allowed to perform the following kicks or throws.

### THROW-IN

If a ball completely crosses a sideline, the team to last touch the ball looses possession and a throw-in is awarded. A goal cannot be scored directly from a throw-in. The thrower cannot touch the ball after a throw-in until another player touches it first.

## GOAL (DEFENSIVE) KICK

When the ball crosses the endline after being touched by an attacking player, a free defensive kick is awarded. The ball is placed anywhere on the line in front of the goal. All players must be at least 5 yards from the ball.

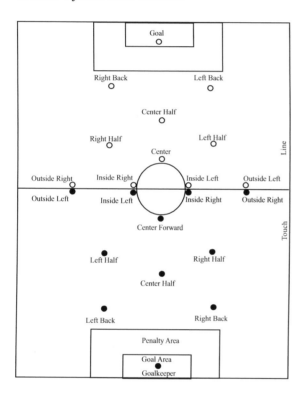

## CORNER KICK

If the defensive team causes the ball to cross the endline, the offensive team is given a corner kick. The ball is placed at the corner of the field (where the sideline and endline meet.) All players must be at least 5 yards from the ball. A goal may be scored from a corner kick.

## Player's Positions

1. Goalkeeper
2. Right Fullback
3. Left Fullback
4. Right Halfback
5. Center Halfback (sweeper)
6. Left Halfback
7. Outside Right Forward
8. Inside Right Forward
9. Center Forward
10. Inside Left Forward
11. Outside Left Forward

## Penalty Rules
### INDIRECT FREE KICK

A goal cannot be scored from an indirect free kick. It is awarded after an offside, holding, or "unsportman-like conduct" penalty is called. The ball is placed where the penalty took place. All players must stand at least five yards from the ball.

### DIRECT FREE KICK

A goal may be scored from a direct free kick. It is awarded after a use of hands, tripping, or pushing penalty. The ball is placed where the penalty took place. All players must stand at least 5 yards from the ball.

### PENALTY KICK

If a use of hands, tripping, or pushing penalty occurs within the penalty box, a penalty kick is awarded. The ball is placed on the 12-yard penalty mark in front of the goal.

### OFFSIDE

A player is offside and loses possession of the ball if he is nearer the opponents' goal than the ball, unless: (1) he is in his own half of the field; (2) there are at least two opponents nearer the goal than he is; or (3) he was the last one to kick the ball.

## Basic Skills
### KICKING
#### Instep Kick
Instruct the students to: (1) approach the ball at a 45-degree angle with two to three steps; (2) plant the left foot beside the ball; (3) contact the ball with the top portion of the ball of the foot; (4) watch the foot contact the rear middle part of the ball.

#### Punting
Instruct the students to: (1) hold the ball with both hands at waist height; (2) place the left foot forward; (3) swing the right leg forward; (4) drop the ball as the leg swings forward; (5) watch the foot contact the ball with the shoelace area of the foot; (6) kick the ball upward at a 45-degree angle.

#### Volley Kick
Instruct the student to kick the ball while it is in the air after it has been thrown or kicked.

### DRIBBLING
Dribbling is moving the ball with short pushes in any direction. If the ball is kicked too far (4 to 5 feet,) an opponent may take possession. Students begin by walking slowly and increasing speed as skill improves. Instruct the students to: (1) stand on their left foot; (2) with the right foot, push the ball forward and to the left; (3) stand on their right foot; (4) with the left foot, push the ball forward and to the right; (5) repeat.

### TRAPPING
Trapping is stopping the ball while it is rolling or in the air.

#### Foot Trap
Instruct the students to: (1) stand on the left foot; (2) have the right foot toes 8 inches off the ground; (3) have the heel lower than the toes; (4) have the ball roll under the toes; (5) when the ball contacts the foot, step down on the ball.

#### Shin Trap
Instruct the students to: (1) stand with feet 4 inches apart; (2) bend the shins forward to a 60-degree angle; (3) after the ball has rolled or bounced into their shins, attempt to take control of the ball.

#### Chest Trap
Instruct the students to: (1) extend their arms to the side; (2) hunch the shoulders forward; (3) lean forward at the waist slightly; (4) allow the ball to contact the sternum bone of the chest; (5) after the ball has dropped to the ground, attempt to gain control of the ball.

### HEADING
Heading is hitting the ball with the forehead. Instruct the students to: (1) stand with one foot in front of the other; (2) watch the ball; (3) have the ball contact the hairline of the forehead; (4) have their arms out to the side for balance; (5) for added force lean forward as they contact the ball.

### THROW-IN
When the ball goes out-of-bounds on the sidelines, it is put back into play with a throw-

in. The rules state that both feet must be touching the ground when the ball leaves the hands. To produce the maximal force in the throw, the students should: (1) hold the sides of the ball with both hands; (2) arch the back backwards; (3) bend the elbows and bring the ball back until it touches the neck; (4) throw the ball forward by extending the elbows and straightening the back.

## TACKLING

Tackling is taking the ball away from your opponent. The rules state that you may not use your hands and you cannot tackle from behind the player. Body contact tackling is legal under men's rules, but I recommend you make contact tackling illegal for your classes. Instruct the students to: (1) watch the ball and not the opponent; (2) when the ball is between you and your opponent, attempt to kick it away from him.

## Sequence of Presenting Skills and Rules

The appropriate skill to teach depends upon what has previously been learned and the ability of the students.

| Rule | Grade |
| --- | --- |
| Goalie use of hands | 1–up |
| Kick-off | 2–up |
| Free kick | 2–up |
| Penalty kick | 2–up |
| Goal (defensive) kick | 3–up |
| Corner kick | 3–up |
| Positions, field markings | 3–up |
| Charging, pushing | 3–up |
| Goalie privileges | 3–up |
| Off side | 4–up |

| Skill | Grade |
| --- | --- |
| Instep kick | K–up |
| Dribbling | K–up |
| Foot trap | 1–up |
| Heading | 1–up |
| Throw-in | 2–up |
| Punting kick | 3–up |
| Volley kick | 3–up |
| Tackling | 3–up |
| Shin trap | 3–up |
| Chest trap | 6–up |

| No. | Activity | Kick | Trap | Dribble | Throw | Grade |
| --- | --- | --- | --- | --- | --- | --- |
| 1. | Foot Trap | x | x | | | K+ |
| 2. | Clean Your Backyard | x | x | x | | K+ |
| 3. | Wall Kick | x | x | | | K+ |
| 4. | Steal | x | x | x | | K+ |
| 5. | Heading | | | | | 1+ |
| 6. | Shuttle Dribble | x | x | x | | K+ |
| 7. | Goal Kick | x | | | | K+ |

| No. | Activity | Kick | Trap | Dribble | Throw | Grade |
|-----|----------|------|------|---------|-------|-------|
| 8. | Goal Run | x | x | x | | K+ |
| 9. | Sideline Soccer | x | x | x | x | K+ |
| 10. | Four Goal Soccer | x | x | x | x | 3+ |
| 11. | Hockey Rink Soccer | x | x | x | x | 3+ |

## Drills and Modified Games

These drills are listed in the approximate order you would present to your students. The easier drills are listed first, followed by the harder or more complex drills. The drills and games may be modified to meet unique limitations of equipment or playing area. Modified goals can be made from common items such as tumbling mats, tape on a wall, cones, milk jugs, and fiberglass bike flags. When the numbers of balls are limited, any type of ball can be used for most drills (8-inch rubber ball, Nerf ball, tennis ball, soccer ball.)

1. **Foot Trap Drill** (K–up)

    Equipment: balls for half the students

    Skills: foot trap, kicking accurately

    Kick a ball gently to a partner. The partner will trap the ball by having his toes higher than his heel and letting the ball roll under his foot. He will then step on the ball to stop it from rolling. Slowly increase the distance to challenge their accuracy.

2. **Clean Your Backyard** (K–up)

    Equipment: 5 to 12 Nerf balls, tennis balls, or rubber playground balls

    Skill: kicking, trapping

    Students are divided into two groups. The mid-court basketball line divides the court into two areas. Team A must stay within its assigned half court and Team B in its assigned half-court. The balls are tossed out and each group tries to kick the balls out of their court into the other team's court. At the end of 2 minutes the whistle is blown and a count is taken of the number of balls on each court. The team with the fewest number of balls gets one point. Only the feet may be used. Repeat.

    Variation: Each team tries to kick balls so they hit the back wall in the opponent's court. One point is awarded for each ball that touches the back wall. At the end of 5 minutes, start over.

3. **Wall-Kicking Drill** (K–up)

    Equipment: 1 ball for each student

    Skill: kicking, trapping

    Students line up approximately 6 feet from a wall with 4 feet between students. Each student kicks the ball into the wall and retrieves the rebound with a foot trap or shin trap.

    Variations: Allow each child to kick the moving rebound.

    Have the student dribble 10 feet to a line and then kick the ball into the wall.

4. **Steal Game** (K–up)

    Equipment: approximately half as many balls as students

    Skill: dribbling, defense

Students who have a ball must dribble it around the area. Students without a ball try to steal a ball. Stop every minute. Students with a ball are awarded one point. Use of the hands is not allowed.

**5. Heading Drill** (1-up)

Equipment: 1 ball per student

Skill: heading

Each student will stand 4 feet from a wall. They will toss the ball 3 to 4 feet above their heads. They will watch the ball come down to their head and head the ball into the wall.

**6. Shuttle Dribble Drill** (K–up)

Equipment: 4 balls, 4 cones

Skill: dribbling

This is a relay race. Divide the students into 4 squads. Place the cones or chairs at midcourt. One player at a time must dribble the ball out to the cone, around the cone twice, and back to the next person in line. The next person does the same. Each team is awarded one point for each person who dribbles out and back. Have them do it continuously for 4 minutes. You will not need to have an equal number of students on each team if you use a time limit.

Variation: Have the student dribble out to the cone and then kick the ball back to the next person in line. After they kick the ball, they return to the end of the line.

**7. Goal Kicking Drill** (K–up)

Equipment: 4 balls, mats or pails or tape to mark goals approximately 6 to 8 feet wide

Skill: kicking accurately, goalie skills

Divide the students into squads of 3 to 6 students each. One student plays goalie while another student kicks the ball from 15

feet way. The goalie goes to the back of the squad line, the kicker becomes goalie, and the next student in line is the kicker.

**8. Goal Run Drill** (K–up)

Equipment: 1 ball for each student, 2 goals marked at opposite ends of the gym.

Skill: kicking accurately, dribbling, goalie skills

Two students play goalie. The rest of the students dribble and must shoot at Goal A from a distance of 10 feet or greater. They keep trying until they score a goal on Goal A. They then dribble to Goal B and keep shooting until they make a goal. Then repeat. Have the students keep track of how many goals they make. Change goalies every 3 minutes until everyone has a chance.

Variation: Add one defensive back to each end to help the goalie defend the goal.

**9.** Sideline Soccer Game (K–up)

Equipment: 2 to 3 balls.

Regular basketball courts are the boundaries.

Skills: all soccer skills

Divide the students into two teams. Assign a number to each member of a team (Mary is 1, Ted is 2, Mark is 3, Jill is 4.) until all students have a number. The students whose number you call (3, 4, 5) will run onto the playing area.

Example: The teacher calls numbers 1,2 or 3. Three players from each team will run onto the court and play the game.

Those students whose numbers were not called must stand out-of-bounds along their assigned side line. If a ball goes out-of-bounds, those students standing out-of-bounds may play it and pass the ball to teammates. Rotate players every 3 to 4 minutes.

Variation: Use two or three balls at the same time. This will give the less skilled players more opportunity to handle the ball. The score ends the play and new numbers are called and fresh players come in. Three or four players per team at a time works best.

10. **Four Goal Soccer** (3–up)

Equipment: 4 balls, 4 goals

Skills: all soccer skills

Divide the class into 4 teams. The goals are placed in the four corners of the playing area. Four or more balls are put into play. Teams try to score on other goals. When a goal is scored, the goalie throws the ball back to midfield or to a teammate. The team with the fewest amount of goals scored on its goal wins.

11. **Hockey Rink Soccer** (3–up)

Equipment: hockey rink with boards or tennis court with fence, 1 ball

Skills: all soccer skills

Playing soccer outdoors in an ice rink allows the students to play and practice the skills more by spending less time chasing the ball. The less skilled players can play more easily.

# LAB: SOCCER KICK
# TECHNIQUE CHECKLIST
### (written for right hander)

Performer's Name _____ Age _____

Perform a soccer kick while someone observes you from the front, side, and back. The observer will look at one item from the checklist at a time and record a yes or no. Did you get "yes" for all the questions? If not, do it again, trying to correct your errors. (Younger children can use a rubber ball.) Videotape the person and have him use this checklist on himself.

## Soccer kick description:

Run up to the ball from the left side from a 45-degree angle in relation to the direction you intend to kick the ball. While keeping the eyes focused on the ball, place the non-kicking foot 4 to 10 inches to the side of the ball with the knee slightly bent. The last step should be longer than previous steps. The body should be slightly leaning away from the kicking foot and the arms are out to the sides for balance. The eyes should focus on a spot slightly below the middle of the ball, and this is where the foot should contact the ball. The contact area of the foot is the area at the base of the big toe.

## I. Legs
### APPROACH

**A.** Is the ball approached from a 45-degree angle?              Yes        No

### FOOT

**B** Is the non-kicking foot planted beside the ball 4 to 8 inches to the side?

　　　　　　　　　　　　　　　　　　　　　　　　　　　　Yes        No
**C.** Does the foot contact the middle of the ball?              Yes        No
**D.** Is the last step longer than the preceding steps?          Yes        No
**E.** Is the ball contacted by the area at the base of the toe and the inside of the foot?              Yes        No

## II. Arms

**A.** Is the body slightly leaning away from the kicking foot?    Yes        No
**B.** Are the arms out to the side for balance?                  Yes        No

## III. Eyes

**A.** Are the eyes focused on the ball?                          Yes        No

**Helpful phrase to say, "Watch the foot hit the center of the ball."**

# LAB: SOCCER HEADING
# TECHNIQUE CHECKLIST

Performer's Name _____ Age _____

    Head a soccer ball while someone observes you from the front, side, and back. The observer will look at one item from the checklist at a time and record a yes or no. Did you get "yes" for all the questions? If not, do it again, trying to correct your errors. (Younger children can use a foam ball.) Videotape the person and have him use this checklist on himself.

## Soccer heading description:

    Lean back with an arch in the back. The arms should be held out to the sides for balance. Move the head forward to meet the ball and focus your eyes on the middle of the ball. The ball should contact the forehead at the hairline. The eyes should be kept open at all times.

## I. Stance

| | | | |
|---|---|---|---|
| **A.** | Is the body facing the ball? | Yes | No |
| **B.** | Is one foot ahead of the other? | Yes | No |
| **C.** | Are the arms out to the sides for balance? | Yes | No |
| **D.** | Is the back slightly arched? | Yes | No |

## II. Contact With the Ball

| | | | |
|---|---|---|---|
| **A.** | Are the eyes always open and watching the ball? | Yes | No |
| **B.** | Does the ball contact the forehead at the hairline? | Yes | No |
| **C.** | Does the whole body move forward from the hips to meet the ball? | Yes | No |

**Helpful phrase to say, "Keep your eyes open."**

# LAB: SOCCER FOOT TRAP
# TECHNIQUE CHECKLIST

Performer's Name _____ Age _____

    Perform a foot trap while someone observes you from the front, side, and back. The observer will look at one item from the checklist at a time and record a yes or no. Did you get "yes" for all the questions? If not, do it again, trying to correct your errors. (Younger children can use a smaller ball.) Videotape the person and have him use this checklist on himself.

## Soccer foot trap description:

    As the ball rolls toward you, raise the right heel 4 to 6 inches off the ground, toes up to form a "V" between the ground and the sole of the foot. Focus the eyes on the ball and watch the ball roll under the foot. Step on the ball lightly to stop its rolling.

## I. Stance

    **A.** Are the arms out to the side for balance?        Yes    No

    **B.** Is the heel off the ground 4 to 6 inches?        Yes    No

    **C.** Is the toe higher than the heel?        Yes    No

## II. Stopping the ball

    **A.** Does the foot step down lightly on the ball?        Yes    No

**Helpful phrase to say, "Step lightly on the ball."**

# LAB: SOCCER DRIBBLING
## TECHNIQUE CHECKLIST
### (written for right hander)

Performer's Name _____ Age _____

    Dribble a ball while someone observes you from the front, side, and back. The observer will look at one item from the checklist at a time and record a yes or no. Did you get "yes" for all the questions? If not, do it again, trying to correct your errors. (Younger children can use a smaller ball.) Videotape the person and have him use this checklist on himself.

## Soccer dribbling description:

    Dribbling in soccer is moving the ball with short pushes with either foot. Because the ball must be in constant control, do not let the ball get more than 4 to 5 feet away from the feet. The skill is developed by very slow walking and increasing the speed of the dribble as the skill improves. Shift your weight to the left foot. Move the ball forward by contacting the ball with the inside of the right foot. Place the right foot down and move the ball forward by contacting the ball with the inside of the left foot. The ball may also be dribbled by making contact with the ball with the outside of the foot at the base of the little toe.

## I. Feet

**A.** Is the ball being hit by the inside of the foot at the base of the toe?

                                                                                 Yes      No

**B.** Does the ball stay within 3 to 6 feet from the foot?        Yes      No

**C.** Is the ball hit with alternate feet?                    Yes      No

**Helpful phrase to say, "Watch the foot hit the ball."**

## FOOTBALL

Parents usually think of football as a contact sport that takes expensive equipment. By modifying the game, it can be a fun noncontact sport for both boys and girls which can be used to teach the skills of throwing and kicking.

## History

Football was invented in the United States in 1869 and was played between Harvard, Yale, Princeton, and Rutgers. It is an American adaptation of the English game rugby. The rules have been modified through the years and today we have regular tackle football and touch/flag football.

## Basic Rules

Touch or flag football teams consist of 7 to 11 players who attempt to advance the ball across the field and across the goal line to score. The game is started by a place kick from the 20-yard line. Teams are given four or five plays to score. If they have not scored in four plays either the defense takes possession of the ball or the offense may punt the ball. The play is dead in flag football when the ball carrier's flag falls off, is detached, or the carrier's knee touches the ground. In touch football, the play is dead when the ball carrier is touched by an opposing player with both hands between the shoulders and knees. A fumbled ball is alive until one team takes possession of it. A fumbled ball may be advanced. No blocking is allowed. A 15-yard penalty is assigned for the following reasons: (1) if both feet of a player leave the ground simultaneously in an attempted block; (2) tripping; or (3) tackling. A 5-yard penalty is assigned if a player is on the opponent's side of the ball when the ball is snapped.

## Basic Skills

- Forward Pass
- Lateral Pass
- Catching
- Punting
- Place Kicking
- Hiking

### LATERAL PASS

A lateral pass must be thrown to a player who is behind the passer. The ball is thrown with two hands, underhanded, and to the side of the passer.

### CATCHING

The ball should be caught with the fingertips and hands. Moving the hands toward the body as the ball is being caught will reduce the chance of the ball rebounding off the hands.

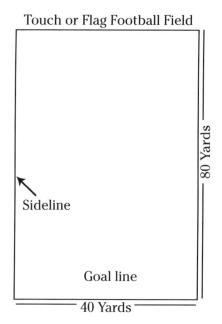
Touch or Flag Football Field

## PUNTING

The ball should be held at waist height with both hands, with the laces up. The arms should be fully extended. Initiate the kick by taking two or three steps forward. Drop the ball (do not toss it) and watch the ball as it contacts the foot. The ball should contact the foot on the area of the shoelaces and slightly to the right of the shoelaces. The leg should kick straight forward and up. The ball should contact the foot when the leg is in a position of 7 o'clock to 8 o'clock.

## PLACE KICKING

The ball is held by a teammate or placed in a tee. The kicker will run straight at the ball, take three to five steps, place the non-kicking foot beside the ball, and watch his toe kick the bottom middle of the football.

## FORWARD PASS

Grip the ball with the index finger in the middle of the ball with fingers on the laces. The body should be facing sideways to the target (perpendicular to the line of scrimmage,) so that the left shoulder is pointing at the target. The ball should be held beside the right ear. The humerus of the throwing arm should be parallel to the ground and elbow the same height as the shoulder. As the throw is initiated, a short step forward is taken with the left foot. The hips and shoulders rotate forward. The ball is kept approximately 2 inches from the ear and the elbow kept at shoulder height throughout the step and rotation. The elbow is extended and the ball released. The arm will follow through after release, down and across the body.

## HIKING

The ball is grasped with both hands, similar to a forward pass. The legs are wide apart and the ball is on the ground in front of the head. The student looks at the receiver between his legs. The ball is hiked or passed between his legs to the receiver. He is to watch the ball until it gets to the receiver's hands.

## Sequence of Presenting Skills

| Skill | Grade |
| --- | --- |
| Forward Pass | 2–up |
| Catching | 2–up |
| Hiking | 2–up |
| Punting | 3–up |
| Place Kicking | 4–up |
| Lateral Pass | 5–up |

## Sequence of Presenting Rules

| Rule | Grade |
| --- | --- |
| Line of Scrimmage | 2–up |
| Number of Downs | 2–up |
| Off Side | 2–up |
| Kick-Off | 3–up |
| Field Markings | 4–up |
| Pass Patterns | 4–up |
| Penalties | 4–up |
| Plays | 4–up |

## Pass Patterns
### HOOK

A pass receiver runs 8 to 10 yards down field, stops, turns and runs back toward the passer. The receiver is moving toward the ball when he catches the ball. The passer throws the ball just as the receiver turns. The path the receiver runs looks like a fish hook. It is very difficult to defend this type of pass.

## SQUARE IN

A pass receiver runs 8 to 10 yards down field, turns a right angle in and runs across the field. The passer then passes the ball. The path the receiver takes looks like a square corner.

## SQUARE OUT

A pass receiver runs 8 to 10 yards down field, turns a right angle out and runs toward the sideline. The passer then passes the ball. The path the receiver takes looks like a square corner.

## ANGLE IN

A pass receiver runs 8 to 10 yards down field, turns a 45-degree angle in and runs across and up the field. The passer then passes the ball. The

path the receiver takes looks like a 45-degree angle.

## ANGLE OUT

A pass receiver runs 8 to 10 yards down field, turns a 45-degree angle out and runs across and up the field toward the sideline. The passer then passes the ball. The path the receiver takes looks like a 45-degree angle.

## POST

The pass receiver runs downfield toward the goal post. The passer then passes the ball.

The ball is thrown the longest distance of any of the passes and is the hardest pass for the receiver to catch.

| No | Activity | Forward Pass | Lateral Pass | Catching | Hiking | Punting | Place Kick | Grade |
|---|---|---|---|---|---|---|---|---|
| 1. | Passing Drill | x | | x | | | | 2–up |
| 2. | Hiking Drill | | | x | x | | | 2–up |
| 3. | File Relay | x | x | x | x | | | 2–up |
| 4. | Pass Pattern Drill | x | | x | | | | 2–up |
| 5. | Punting Drill | | | x | | x | | 2–up |
| 6. | Place Kicking Drill | | | | | | x | 2–up |
| 7. | Pass Defense Drill | x | | x | | | | 3–up |
| 8. | 500 Football | | | x | | x | | 1–up |
| 9. | Ultimate Football | x | | x | | | | 3–up |
| 10. | Punt & Catch | | | | x | x | | 3–up |
| 11. | Flag Football | x | x | x | x | x | x | 4–up |

## Drills and Modified Games

**1. Passing Drill**

Equipment: 1 ball per pair

Skills: passing, catching

Students are paired and stand in two parallel lines 10 feet apart. Pass the ball back and forth. Have the lines move further apart as skill increases.

**2. Hiking Drill**

Equipment: 1 ball per pair

Skills: hiking

Students are paired and stand in two parallel lines 10 feet apart. Hike the ball back and forth. Have the lines move further apart as skill increases.

**3. File Relay**

Equipment: 1 ball per 3 to 5 students

Skill: passing

The first student on each team runs with the ball 12 to 20 feet to a line, turns around, and throws the ball to the next player in line. After the ball is thrown, the player runs to the end of his line. For competition, have teams count how many passes they catch.

Variation: Shorten the distance and require a hike or lateral pass.

Player A runs to the line without the ball and Player B, from the start line, throws the ball to him. When the ball is caught he must run back to his line and hand off to Player C who throws to B. A goes to the back of his team's line after the handoff.

**4. Pass Patterns Drill**

Equipment: 1 ball per pair

Skills: passing, catching, pass patterns

Students are paired. One student is the passer and the other student runs a pass pattern called by the teacher. The passer and receiver change positions. All students run the same pass pattern at the same time on the instructor's command (hook, square in, square out, angle in, angle out, post).

Variation: A timed race—count the number of passes a pair catches in one minute.

**5. Punting Drill**

Equipment: 1 ball per pair

Skills: punting

Students are paired and stand in two parallel lines 20 feet apart. Punt the ball back and forth. Have the lines move farther apart as skill increases.

**6. Place Kick Drill**

Equipment: 1 ball per pair

Skills: place kick

Students are paired. One student holds the ball while the partner kicks the ball. The kicker retrieves the ball and the holder becomes the kicker.

**7. Pass Defense Drill**

Equipment: 1 ball for 3 students

Skills: passing, catching, defense, patterns

Students are in groups of three. One student is the defense, one the receiver, and one the passer. The passer tells the receiver which pattern to run. The defense tries to intercept or bat down the pass. Rotation is from passer to receiver, receiver to defense, defense to passer.

**8. 500 Football**

Equipment: 1 ball per game

Skill: punting, catching

A player is appointed as punter. The punter punts the ball into the air to a group of players downfield. If a player successfully catches the ball, he is awarded points: 100

points for a fly, 50 points for one bounce, 25 points for two bounces, 10 points for a rolling ball. If a player touches a ball and is unsuccessful in catching the ball, he is awarded negative points. For example, a player who drops a fly ball is awarded a negative 100 points and a player behind him who catches the ball on one bounce is awarded 50 points. The first player to score 500 is the new thrower.

Variation: kick a rubber utility ball (grades 1–2) or football (grades 3–up)

## 9. Ultimate Football

Equipment: 1 ball per game, cones to mark boundaries

Skills: passing, catching, patterns, aerobic

Formation: 4 to 8 students per team

Divide into two teams. Establish two goal lines. The goal is to get the football across the opponent's goal line by throwing the football to a teammate. The person throwing the football must remain stationary. If the football touches the ground, the other team takes possession of it. The football may be intercepted. A tennis or Nerf ball can be substituted for a football for younger players.

Defense

One-on-one with ball

One-on-one without ball 2–up

## 10. Football Punt and Catch

Equipment: 1 ball per game, cones to mark boundaries

Skills: catching, punting accurately

Mark three zones on a field, each approximately 20 feet square. The middle zone is the neutral zone. Divide into two teams. Team A punts the ball. If

the ball lands or is caught in Team B's zone, then Team A gets a point. If Team B catches the ball, Team B also gets a point. Team B then punts the ball back to Team A. (Grades 3 to 6) Two or more players.

## 11. Flag Football

Equipment: 1 ball per game, flags (colored rags,) cones

Skills: all

Formation: 4 to 8 students per team

This is regular football except instead of tackling the ball carrier, pulling off one of the ball carrier's flags is equal to a tackle. All students have two flags tucked in their belts. Teams are given five plays to score. If they have not scored in four plays, the defense takes possession of the ball. The play is dead when one of the ball carrier's flags falls off, is detached, or the carrier's knee touches the ground. No blocking is allowed. Defensive players may detach only the ball carrier's flag which is returned after the play is dead.

Variation: No running with the ball is allowed. Passing only. The defense may not rush the passer.

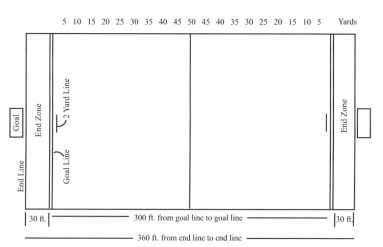

# LAB: FOOTBALL PASSING TECHNIQUE CHECKLIST
### (written for right hander)

Performer's Name _____ Age _____

    Perform a football pass while someone observes you from the front, side and back. The observer will look at one item from the checklist at a time and record a yes or no. Did you get "yes" for all the questions? If not, do it again, trying to correct your errors. (Younger children can use a small Nerf football.) Videotape the person and have him use this checklist on himself.

## Football pass description:

    Grip the ball with the index finger in the middle of the ball with fingers on the laces. The body should be facing sideways to the target (perpendicular to the line of scrimmage.) so that the left shoulder is pointing at the target. The ball should be held beside the right ear. The upper arm should be parallel to the ground and elbow the same height as the shoulder. As the throw is initiated, a short step forward is taken with the left foot. The hips and shoulders rotate forward. The ball is kept approximately 2 inches from the ear and the elbow kept at shoulder height through-out the step and rotation. The elbow is extended and the ball released. The arm will follow through after release, down and across the body.

## I. Grip

|  |  |  |
|---|---|---|
| **A.** Is the ball held in the fingers and not the palm? | Yes | No |
| **B.** Are the fingers about half an inch apart? | Yes | No |
| **C.** Is the little finger placed on the laces near the middle of the ball? | Yes | No |
| **D.** Is the index finger 1 inch behind the last lace? | Yes | No |
| **E.** Is the thumb on the bottom of the ball? | Yes | No |

## II. Stance

|  |  |  |
|---|---|---|
| **A.** Are the feet shoulder width apart? | Yes | No |
| **B.** Is a majority of the weight on the back foot? | Yes | No |
| **C.** Are the feet perpendicular to the line of scrimmage? | Yes | No |
| **D.** Are the left shoulder and hip pointing to the target? | Yes | No |
| **E.** Is the non-throwing arm closest to the target? | Yes | No |
| **F.** Is the ball held at the ear? | Yes | No |
| **G.** Is the elbow high and arm parallel with the ground? | Yes | No |

|  |  | Yes | No |
|---|---|---|---|
| **H.** | Is the trunk erect? | Yes | No |
| **I.** | Is the head up, erect, and eyes focused on the target? | Yes | No |

## III. Delivery

**A.** Is a short step taken with the front foot toward the line of scrimmage?

|  |  | Yes | No |
|---|---|---|---|
|  | | Yes | No |
| **B.** | Is the weight shifted from the rear to front foot? | Yes | No |
| **C.** | Is the front foot pointed in the direction of the intended target? | | |
|  | | Yes | No |
| **D.** | Do the hips rotate until the body is facing the target? | Yes | No |
| **E.** | Do the shoulders rotate until the body is facing the target? | Yes | No |
| **F.** | Is the ball kept near the ear during the throw? | Yes | No |
| **G.** | Is the ball brought forward by forcefully extending the elbow? | Yes | No |
| **H.** | Is the forearm brought forward perpendicular to the ground? | Yes | No |
| **I.** | Does the elbow remain at shoulder height throughout the throw? | Yes | No |
| **J.** | Is the index finger the last finger to leave the ball? | Yes | No |
| **K.** | At the moment of release of the ball, is the elbow of the throwing arm almost fully extended? | Yes | No |
| **L.** | Do the eyes remain fixed on the target? | Yes | No |

# LAB: FOOTBALL PUNT
# TECHNIQUE CHECKLIST
### (written for right hander)

Performer's Name _____ Age _____

   Perform a football pass while someone observes you from the front, side, and back. The observer will look at one item from the checklist at a time and record a yes or no. Did you get "yes" for all the questions? If not, do it again, trying to correct your errors. (Younger children can use a small Nerf football.) Videotape the person and have him use this checklist on himself.

## Football punt description:

   The ball should be held at waist height with both hands, with the laces up. The arms should be fully extended. Initiate the kick by taking two or three steps forward. Drop the ball (do not toss it) and watch the ball as it contacts the foot. The ball should contact the foot on the area of the shoe laces and slightly to the right of the laces. The leg should kick straight forward and up. The ball should contact the foot when the leg is in a position of 7 o'clock to 8 o'clock.

## I. BALL

**A.** Is the ball held at waist height by both hands?     Yes     No
**B.** Are the arms straight?     Yes     No
**C.** Is the ball dropped and not thrown up in the air?     Yes     No
**D.** Is the ball contacted with the outside edge of the shoe laces?

     Yes     No
**E.** Are the eyes focused on the ball during the kick?     Yes     No
**F.** Is the flight of the ball (leaving the foot) between 45 and 60 degrees?

     Yes     No

## II. LEG

**A.** Does the leg swing straight forward and up?     Yes     No
   (The leg should not swing sideways.)

**Helpful phrase to say, "Watch the ball hit the shoelaces."**

## BASKETBALL

### History

Basketball was invented in the United States in 1891 by the YMCA. It quickly gained popularity and is played all around the world today. Indoor and outdoor courts are abundant today with many homes having a hoop in the driveway. Basketball should be considered a basic activity for a physical education program because: (1) it is widely played by all ages in the U.S.; (2) many components of physical education are involved in the game (aerobics, ball skills); (3) the game can be easily modified for varying court sizes and skill levels of players; (4) courts are easily accessible; and (5) equipment costs per student are very low.

### Basic Rules

Teams consist of five players with unlimited substitution of players. The game begins with a jump ball at midcourt. Players move the ball among themselves by passing, dribbling with the intent of scoring by putting the ball through the hoop, and trying to prevent the opponents from scoring. You can prevent highly skilled players from dominating the play by modification of the rules, such as lowering basket height, limiting the number of dribbles, and requiring a minimum number of passes.

#### SCORING

Two points are awarded for each field goal and one point for each free throw. Three points are awarded for field goals made beyond a certain distance from the basket. (The three-point rule tends to reduce the amount of teamwork and for instructional purposes, I suggest you use the three-point rule.)

#### VIOLATIONS

When a violation is committed the ball is awarded to the other team.

- **a.** Traveling—a player takes more than one step with the ball without dribbling.
- **b.** Double dribbling—a player dribbles the ball, stops, then dribbles again.
- **c.** Kicking the ball—kicking the ball with the foot or leg.
- **d.** Lane violation—offensive players are only allowed to stand within the free throw area for 3 seconds.
- **e.** Five-second violation—throwing in the ball from out-of-bounds must be done within the 5 second time limit.
- **f.** Over and back—once a team has advanced the ball across the midcourt line, they may not cross the line into the backcourt.

#### FOULS

A player is charged with a foul if he commits unsportsmanlike conduct, holds, charges, trips, or pushes another player.

- **a.** If a player is fouled in the act of shooting, he is awarded two free throws.
- **b.** A fifth personal foul sidelines the player for the rest of the game.

### Skills
#### OUTLINE OF BASKETBALL SKILLS

Passing

Chest Pass

Two-hand bounce pass

One-hand bounce pass

Overhead pass

Baseball pass

Catching

Dribbling
Shooting
Lay-up
Free throw
Jump shot
Hook shot
Pivot

## TWO-HAND CHEST PASS

Stand with both feet together and hold the ball so it touches the chest and is a couple of inches below the chin. Focus the eyes on the target. Take one step forward and at the same time push the ball forward. The pass should end with the palms facing outward and the thumbs pointing down. A common error is for the child to throw harder with the dominant arm. Both arms must be used equally.

## BOUNCE PASS

Focus the eyes on a spot two-thirds the distance between you and the other person. Do a two-hand chest pass to that spot. The ball will bounce to the receiver's waist height.

## DRIBBLING

The ball should be contacted with the fingertips and be bounced waist high.

## LAY-UP

Approach the basket at a 45-degree angle from the right side. Raise the right knee up and bring the ball up with both hands. Continue jumping up and shoot the ball with the right hand. Shoot the ball into the square on the backboard and it will rebound into the basket.

## FREE THROW

Focus the eyes on the hole in the basket. Place the right foot in front of the left. Hold the ball near the chin. Have the wrist, elbow, and shoulder in a vertical plane with the basket. Straighten the knees and push the ball forward with the arm. The fingers should point to the basket at the end of the shot.

## PIVOT

With weight on the ball of the right foot, move the left foot in any direction.

## DEFENSIVE SKILLS

1. Stay between the man you are guarding and the basket.
2. When guarding a person with the ball, focus the eyes on his or her waist and keep your hands below your waist.
3. When trying to steal the ball, always slap up at the ball.

# Suggested Sequence of Presenting Skills

| Skill | Grade |
|---|---|
| **Passing** | |
| Two-hand chest pass | 1–up |
| Two-hand bounce pass | 2–up |
| Overhead pass | 2–up |
| One hand bounce pass | 3–up |
| Baseball pass | 3–up |
| **Dribbling** | |
| Standing dribble | K–up |
| Running dribble | 1–up |
| Changing hands | 3–up |
| Shooting | 1–up |
| Free throw | 3–up |
| Lay-up | 4–up |

| Skill | Grade |
|-------|-------|
| Hook shot | 7–up |
| Jump shot | 3–up |
| Pivot | 3–up |

| Rules presented | Grade |
|-----------------|-------|
| Pick-and-roll | 4–up |
| Offensive charging | 5–up |
| Holding | 3–up |
| Blocking | 5–up |

## Suggested Sequence of Presenting Rules of Basketball

| Rules presented | Grade |
|-----------------|-------|
| Out-of-bounds | 1–up |
| Positions | 2–up |
| 5-second lane | 4–up |
| Traveling | 1–up |
| Double dribble | 3–up |
| Over-and-back | 4–up |
| Scoring | 2–up |
| Give-and-go | 3–up |

### BALL SIZES AND BASKET HEIGHTS RECOMMENDED
- Nerf Ball age 4–6, junior-size ball age 7–9, girl's-size ball age 10–12
- Men's-size ball age 12–up
- Basket height: 6' age 5–6, 7' age 7–9, 8' age 10–11, 9' age 12, 10' age 13–up

## Drills and Modified Games

| No. | Drills and Games | Catching | Passing | Shooting | Dribbling | Pivot | Grades |
|-----|------------------|----------|---------|----------|-----------|-------|--------|
| 1. | Beanbag Basketball | | | x | | | K–up |
| 2. | 5-Gallon Pail | x | x | x | x | | K–up |
| 3. | One Knee Dribbling | | | | x | | K–up |
| 4. | Wall Passing | | x | | | | K–up |
| 5. | Steal | | | | x | | 1–up |
| 6. | Man in the Middle | x | x | | | | K–6 |
| 7. | Relay—one | x | x | | x | x | 1–up |
| 8. | Relay—two | x | x | x | x | | 1–up |
| 9. | Horse | | | x | | | 1–up |
| 10. | Lightning | | | x | x | | 3–up |
| 11. | Twenty-one | x | x | x | | | 3–up |
| 12. | Sideline Basketball | x | x | x | x | x | 4–up |
| 13. | No-Dribble Basketball | x | x | x | | x | 4–up |

## 1. Beanbag Basketball

Equipment: 8 to 20 beanbags, tennis balls or Nerf balls

3 to 5 trash cans or five-gallon plastic pails

Skill: shooting

Students K through 2 can practice their shooting technique by shooting beanbags into trash cans or 5-gallon pails. Divide students into teams of 3 to 5 students per team. Have them stand 10 feet from the pail and shoot using correct free throw technique. The shooter retrieves his own shot, passes the ball to the next student in line, and runs to the end of the line. Have a contest to see how many baskets a team can make in 2 minutes. An excellent drill for when equipment and facilities are lacking. It can be done in a class room.

## 2. Five-Gallon Pail Basketball

Equipment: 2 chairs or tables, 1 to 6 balls (basketball, Nerf ball, tennis ball, or 8" rubber ball)

Skill: all skills

Divide the students into two teams. One player of Team A stands on a chair or table holding a plastic five-gallon pail. His teammates try to shoot the ball into the pail. The student holding the pail may move the pail to help a shot go in. A circle 10 feet in diameter is drawn (chalk or tape) around the pail person. No players are allowed to stand in this area. Team B has a pail person on the opposite end of the playing area. Basketball rules are used: (1) you may not walk while holding the ball; (2) the ball is advanced by dribbling and passing; (3) no pushing or holding. More than five players on a team is allowed. An excellent game when facilities are lacking. The team with the greatest number of baskets in the time limit wins.

Variation: Play with 3 to 8 balls at the same time. The greater number of balls allows more students to participate in the game.

## 3. One-Knee Dribbling

Equipment: 1 ball per student (basketball or 8" rubber ball)

Skill: dribbling

Students place one knee on the ground and dribble the ball back and forth from the right side of the body to the left.

## 4. Wall-Passing Drill

Equipment: 1 ball per student (basketball or 8" rubber ball)

Skill: passing, catching

Players line up approximately 5 feet from the wall and increase the distance as their skill increases. Each player has a ball. All types of passes can be practiced. To work on accuracy, have a line or target on the wall. Have a contest of how many passes they can throw and catch in 60 seconds.

## 5. Steal Game

Equipment: balls for approximately 60% of the students (basketball or rubber ball)

Skill: dribbling, defense

Give balls to 60% of the players. Those without a ball must steal one. Those with a ball must stay in-bounds on half a basketball court. They must dribble the ball (no holding a ball.)

## 6. Man-in-the-Middle Drill

Equipment: 1 ball per 4 to 5 students (basketball or rubber ball)

Skill: passing, catching

Three or four students are in a circle

approximately 10 feet in diameter. One student is in the middle. Outside players are not allowed to move their feet. If the middle player touches the ball or an outside player can not catch a ball, a new middle player is appointed. If the players rotate into the middle in clockwise order, everyone will get equal opportunity to be in the middle. The length of time a person can be in the middle is 60 seconds.

**7. Relay—one**

Equipment: 1 ball per 3 to 5 students (basketball or rubber ball)

Skill: dribbling, pivoting, passing

Divide students into 3 to 5 teams. Each team has one ball. The first player in line dribbles to midcourt, stops, pivots, and throws a pass back to the next teammate in line. He then returns to the end of his line. Teams count how many passes are caught in 2 minutes.

**8. Relay—two**

Equipment: 1 ball per 3 to 5 students (basketball or rubber ball)

Skill: dribble, lay-up, free throw

Divide students into 3 to 5 teams. Each team has one ball. The first player in line dribbles to the far basket and shoots until he makes a lay-up. He then shoots until he makes a free throw. He dribbles to the team and hands the ball to next teammate. One point is awarded for each basket made. The team with the most baskets in 2 minutes wins.

**9. Horse**

Equipment: 1 ball per 2 to 4 students

Skill: shooting

The players determine a rotational order to take turns shooting. The first Player A may shoot from any place in the court. If he misses the shot, then the next Player B may shoot from any place on the court. If Player A makes the shot, Player B must shoot from the same location. If Player B misses, he is given an H. He is assigned a letter for each shot he misses until his score spells horse. If Player B makes his shot, then Player C must shoot from the same location.

**10. Lightning Basketball**

Equipment: 2 balls per 3 to 10 students (basketball, Nerf ball, or rubber ball)

Skill: shooting

Player A and Player B both have a basketball. Player A shoots a free throw and keeps shooting until he makes a basket. After the ball has left Player A's hands, Player B may shoot at the basket. If Player B gets his ball in the basket before Player A, then Player A is eliminated. When Player A makes a basket, he then passes the ball to Player C standing on the free throw-line. Player C tries to make a basket before Player B makes a basket. Repeat until only one player remains.

**11. Twenty-one**

Equipment: 1 basketball per 2 to 14 students (basketball or rubber ball)

Skill: all skills

Players:

Variation one: 2 to 4 players with each playing as his own team.

Variation two: 2 teams play half court with 2 to 7 players on a team.

Rules:

1. Player number one of Team A

shoots a free throw while the other players stand wherever they wish.

2. Player number one continues shooting free throws until he misses. One point is awarded with each made free throw.

3. When a player misses a free throw, any player who gets the ball may try for a field goal or pass to a teammate for a field goal. A field goal counts two points.

4. If the attempted field goal is missed, any team who gets possession may attempt a field goal until a goal is made.

5. After a field goal is made, player one of Team B attempts a free throw.

6. Continue the process until one player or team has twenty-one points.

## 12. Sideline Basketball

Equipment: 1 ball for class

Skill: all skills

1. Five players from each team play on the playing court. The rest of Team A stands along the right sideline and Team B stands along the left sideline. A variation is to allow the teams to have out-of-bounds players standing along both basket sidelines also.

2. Basketball rules are followed except the ball may be passed to teammates on the sideline.

3. When the defensive team takes possession of the ball (by interception of a pass or the other team scores) they must pass the ball to a minimum of one player on the side line before they can score.

## 13. No-Dribble Basketball

Equipment: 1 basketball per 6 to 10 students

Skill: passing, shooting

Regular basketball is modified so that no player may dribble the ball. This drill works on passing skills and learning how to move to be open to receive a pass.

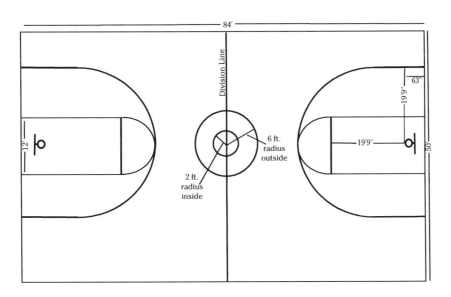

# LAB: BASKETBALL FREE THROW TECHNIQUE CHECKLIST
## (written for right hander)

Performer's Name _____ Age _____

    Shoot a free throw, while someone observes you from the front, side, and back. The observer will look at one item from the checklist at a time and record a yes or no. Did you get "yes" for all the questions? If not, shoot again, trying to correct your errors. (Younger children can shoot a beanbag or small ball into a trash can.) Videotape the shooter and have him use this checklist on himself.

## Free throw description:

Place the right foot slightly in front of the left foot. Hold the ball with both hands in front of the chin. Keep the back straight and the knees in a slightly bent position. The wrist, elbow, and shoulder should be in the same vertical plane pointing to the basket. Simultaneously, straighten the knees and extend the arms forward and upward pushing the ball toward the basket. Release the ball with a slight snap of the wrist and fingers. The ball should have a slight backspin if you snap the wrist correctly. The index finger should be pointing to the basket. The eyes should be focused on the hoop at all times.

## I. STANCE AND PREPARATION
### FEET

| | | |
|---|---|---|
| **A.** Is the right foot 6 to 12 inches ahead of the left foot? | Yes | No |
| **B.** Are the feet shoulder width apart? | Yes | No |
| **C.** Are the feet pointed toward the basket? | Yes | No |
| **D.** Are the hips and knees slightly flexed? | Yes | No |

### HANDS

| | | |
|---|---|---|
| **E.** Is the ball close to the body near the shoulder or face? | Yes | No |
| **F.** Is the non-shooting hand on the side of the ball? | Yes | No |
| **G.** Is the shooting hand in the middle of the ball on the back? | Yes | No |
| **H.** Are the shoulder, elbow, and wrist in a straight vertical line? | Yes | No |

### EYES

| | | |
|---|---|---|
| **I.** Are eyes focused on the middle of the hole (center of the rim)? | | |
| | Yes | No |

## II. SHOT ACTION
### FEET AND LEGS

**A.** Are the hips and knees extending during the shot?  Yes    No

### HANDS

**B.** Is the ball released off the fingertips of the shooting hand?  Yes    No
(evidenced by a back spin on ball)

**C.** Do the shooting hand fingers point to the middle of the basket?
Yes    No

**D.** Do the wrist, elbow, and shoulder remain in a straight vertical line?
Yes    No

## III. ANGLE OF SHOT ENTERING HOOP

**A.** Does the ball enter the hoop at approximately a 45-degree angle?
(a minimum angle of entry for a free throw is 31.5 degrees.)  Yes    No

**Helpful phrase to say, "Focus your eyes on the rim hole,
that is where you want to ball to go."**

# LAB: BASKETBALL LAY-UP
## TECHNIQUE CHECKLIST
### (written for right hander)

Performer's Name _____ Age _____

    Shoot a lay-up while someone observes you from the front, side, and back. The observer will look at one item from the checklist at a time and record a yes or no. Did you get "yes" for all the questions? If not, shoot again, trying to correct your errors. (Younger children can shoot a beanbag or small ball into a trash can.) Videotape the shooter and have him use this checklist on himself.

## Lay-up description:

    Approach the basket from the side at a 45-degree angle, simultaneously shift the weight to the left foot, and raise the ball upward as far as possible with both hands. Release the left hand and carry the ball upward with the right hand. Continue upward with the right hand and lay the ball against the backboard about 12 inches above the rim inside the square. The ball should rebound into the basket.

## I. Preparation
### EYES

**A.** Are eyes focused on the backboard about 6 to 8 inches above
the rim?                                                         Yes       No

### FEET AND HANDS

**B.** Is the left foot planted approximately 3 to 4 feet in front of the
basket and 2 to 3 feet to the right of the middle of the rim?     Yes       No

**C.** Is the ball held firmly with both hands approximately
waist high?                                                       Yes       No

## II. Shot Action
### LEGS

**A.** Does the right knee rise during the shot?            Yes       No

**B.** Is the right thigh approximately parallel to the floor?     Yes       No

**C.** Is the ball raised from waist height to head height?      Yes       No

### HANDS

**D.** Is the right hand behind the ball when the ball is head height?
                                                              Yes       No

**E.** Is the ball released from the fingertips?           Yes       No
(evidenced by backward rotation of the ball)

### BALL

**F.** Does the ball strike the backboard 6 to 8 inches above the rim?
                                                              Yes       No

**Helpful phrase to say, "Focus your eyes on the backboard square."**

# LAB: BASKETBALL TWO-HAND CHEST PASS TECHNIQUE CHECKLIST

Performer's Name _____ Age _____

    Perform a two-hand chest pass while someone observes you from the front, side, and back. The observer will look at one item from the checklist at a time and record a yes or no. Did you get "yes" for all the questions? If not, shoot again, trying to correct your errors. Videotape the passer and have him use this checklist on himself.

## Chest pass description:

    The ball is held close to the chest in both hands, with the elbows out. As you step forward, the arms extend fully and the ball is released. At the point of release, the thumbs should be pointing down with the palms out. Taking a longer step will increase the force of the throw.

## I. Preparation
### FEET
    **A.** Are feet shoulder width apart?               Yes     No

### HANDS
    **B.** Are hands on the sides of the ball?          Yes     No
    **C.** Is the ball touching the chest?            Yes     No

### ELBOWS
    **D.** Are elbows high?                         Yes     No

### EYES
    **E.** Are eyes focused on the receiver's chest?    Yes     No

## II. PASS ACTION
### FEET
    **A.** Is the player stepping forward (either foot) in the direction of the pass?
                                             Yes     No
    **B.** Is the player stepping forward 1 to 3 feet during the pass?   Yes   No
    **C.** Is the player stepping forward in time?     Yes   No
        (stepping as the ball is passed)

### HANDS
    **D.** Is the ball released from the fingertips?     Yes   No
    **E.** Are the thumbs pointed down and palms out after the pass?   Yes   No
    **F.** Are the fingers pointing to the receiver's chest?   Yes   No
    **G.** Is the player passing with both arms equally?   Yes   No

**Helpful phrase to say, "Focus your eyes on the target you want to hit, the person's chest."**

# LAB: BASKETBALL DRIBBLING
# TECHNIQUE CHECKLIST

Performer's Name _____ Age _____

    Dribble while someone observes you from the front, side, and back. The observer will look at one item from the checklist at a time and record a yes or no. Did you get "yes" for all the questions? If not, dribble again, trying to correct your errors. (Younger children use a rubber ball.) Videotape the performer and have him use this checklist on himself.

## Dribbling description:

    The fingers should be spread over the top of the ball. The fingertips should touch the ball. Extend the forearm downward and slightly snap the wrist to dribble the ball down. Hold the hand down and wait for the ball to rebound back. Let the fingers, wrist, and arm ride back with the ball. The ball should be dribbled at waist height with only one hand.

## I. DRIBBLING ACTION
### EYES

    **A.** Are eyes on the playing area and not on the ball?      Yes     No

### HANDS

    **B.** Is the ball contacting the fingertips?      Yes     No
    **C.** Is the hand on top of the ball?      Yes     No
    (error would be carrying the ball)

### BALL

    **D.** Is the ball contacting the floor 2 to 3 inches outside the
        shoulder?      Yes     No
    **E.** Is the ball contacting the floor ahead of the player
        1 to 3 feet?      Yes     No
    **F.** Is the ball raising to waist height?      Yes     No

**Helpful phrase to say, "Feel the ball with your fingertips."**

# SOFTBALL

## History

Softball was invented by the YMCA about 1900. By playing with a softer ball, it could be played in a smaller area and was safer for young children. Softball/baseball are played widely throughout the world by all ages. Softball should be considered a basic activity for a physical education program because: (1) it is widely played by all ages in the U.S.; (2) many components of physical education are involved in the game (striking, catching, throwing); (3) the game can be easily modified for varying field sizes and skill levels of players; (4) only an open grass field is needed, and regular fields are easily accessible; and (5) equipment costs per student are low and most students own their own gloves.

## Basic Rules
### BATTING

The batter is out when: (1) he has three strikes; (2) he is thrown out at first; (3) he is tagged before reaching first; (4) he hits a fly ball that is caught; (5) he interferes with the catcher while he is catching a fly ball or tagging a runner; (6) when a foul ball is caught above the catcher's head.

### RUNNING BASES

The batter advances to first base when he: (1) hits a fair ball and reaches first base before the ball; (2) is walked by four balls called; (3) is hit by a pitch; (4) is interfered with by the catcher while batting (bat hitting the catcher's mitt.)

The base runner when traveling the bases: (1) may advance to the next base after a caught fly ball; (2) may attempt to steal a base after the ball leaves the pitcher's hand; (3) must advance when forced by another base runner; (4) may advance on a fair ball that has not been caught or that has touched the ground.

### PLAYING FIELD

The bases are 60 feet apart. The pitcher's mound is 40 feet from home plate for women and 46 feet for men's fast pitch.

### TYPES OF SOFTBALL

There are two forms of softball: slow pitch and fast pitch. The two main differences are:

♦ In slow pitch, a pitched ball must describe an arc, peaking between 6 and 12 feet.

♦ Slow pitch softball requires one more player than fast pitch (or baseball)—an additional outfielder, for a total of 10 players.

## Basic Skills
### OVERHAND THROW

The left side of the body is facing the direction of the throw. A short step forward is taken with the left foot. The elbow is at the same height as the shoulder. Twist the body (shoulders and hips) to the left as the arm swings forward. After the ball is released, step forward with the right foot. (A common error of young children is to have the wrong foot forward.)

### BATTING

Select a bat that is appropriate to the age. Use an oversized plastic bat for ages 4 to 6. Use a short, light bat for ages 7 to 9. (Cut 4 to 5 inches off the end of a standard wood bat.) Stand with the left side toward the pitcher, with legs shoulder width apart. Grip the bottom of the handle with the left hand below the right hand and the hands touching. Both elbows should be 2 to 5 inches below the shoulder height and the bat held near the right shoulder. The bat should be vertical. After the ball is pitched, take a short step forward with the left foot. (If a child steps to the side instead of toward the pitcher, place a bench behind his legs. This will force him to step forward.) Rotate the hips and shoulders toward the pitcher. Swing the bat forward, keeping your eyes focused on the ball. The right heel will raise off the ground. After contacting the ball, continue to let the swing follow through and drop the bat (do not throw a bat.) The hips and shoulders should be facing the pitcher.

### UNDERHAND PITCH

Stand facing the batter. Hold the ball in front of the body with the right hand. Swing the right hand down and backward until the hand is approximately the same height as the shoulder. The hips and shoulders will be twisted sideways. Swing the arm down and forward. At the same time rotate the hips and shoulders forward and the left foot will step forward. The ball is released and the arm should end pointing to the batter.

| Skill | Grade |
| --- | --- |
| Overhand throw | K–up |
| Underhand pitch | K–up |
| Catching | K–up |
| T-batting | K–up |
| Waffle-pitched batting | 1–up |
| Softball-pitched batting | 2–up |
| Fielding fly balls | 3–up |
| Bunt | 4–up |
| Slide | 4–up |

| Rule | Grade |
| --- | --- |
| Outs by fly | 1–up |
| Outs by touch | 1–up |
| Base running rules | 1–up |
| Force-outs | 2–up |
| Player positions | 2–up |
| Strike zone | 3–up |
| Third strike rule | 3–up |
| Walks | 3–up |
| Infield fly rule | 5–up |

## The Players

Substitutions may take place anytime that the ball is not in play. Once substituted, however, a player may not re-enter the game.

**Pitcher**—Throws the softball from the center of the diamond. Facing the batter, with both feet on the "pitching plate" and both hands on the ball, the pitcher uses an underarm motion to fast pitch the ball toward the "strike zone." While releasing the softball toward home plate, he or she may step forward off the pitching plate, but must keep his or her back foot on the pitching plate until the ball has left her hand. After making the pitch, the pitcher gets ready to field balls hit up the middle of the infield.

**Catcher**—Plays in a semi-crouched position directly behind home plate and catches the ball thrown by the pitcher. He or she also covers home plate on fielding plays when runners try to score.

**First Baseman**—Positioned just to the left of the first base bag. His or her main roles are to make fielding plays on balls hit toward first base and to cover the base on "force plays" when batters approach.

**Second Baseman**—Plays in the gap between the bag at second and the first baseman. He or she fields "grounders" and "pop ups" hit to this side of the infield, covers second when runners approach, and relays throws from the outfielders.

**Shortstop**—Plays between second and third base and fields the balls hit to this area of the infield. He or she covers second base (along with the second baseman) and is often involved in force plays and "double plays" with the second baseman.

**Third Baseman**—Plays to the left of third base and covers any plays there. He or she is responsible for fielding softballs hit down the third base line.

**Outfielders (Left, Right, and Center)**—Positioned beyond the infield, they catch and field "fly balls," line drives, and ground balls hit into the outfield. They usually have strong throwing arms to quickly get the ball back to the infield and prevent runners from advancing.

## Drills and Modified Games

I recommend, during instruction, using a kitten ball or mush ball (oversized and softer softball) or tennis balls. These will allow the students to practice without gloves and it hurts less when a ball hits a student. If a younger student is struck by a regular ball, they may not participate because they are afraid of the ball. Rugs, gymnastic mats, and pails may be used as bases.

| No. | Activity | Throwing | Catching | Batting | Base Running | Grade |
|---|---|---|---|---|---|---|
| 1. | Line Throwing | x | x | | | K–up |
| 2. | Wall Throwing Drill | x | | | | K–up |
| 3. | Mat Kickball | x | x | | x | K–up |
| 4. | Fielding Drill | | x | | | 2–up |
| 5. | T-ball | x | x | x | x | K–1 |
| 6. | Waffle Ball | x | x | x | x | 1–5 |
| 7. | Work-up | x | x | x | x | 4–up |

**1. Line Throwing**

Equipment: Balls for half the class
Skill: throwing, catching
Pair students and have them throw to each other from 20 feet.

**2. Wall Throw Drill**

Equipment: tennis balls, 1 for each student
Skill: throwing accuracy

Have the students throw at a target on the wall.

Variation: Tape a strike zone to the wall and have students pitch to the target.

**3. Mat Kickball**

Equipment: 1 ball, bases 20 to 30 feet apart depending upon age and facility
Skills: kicking, catching, fielding, throwing, teaches the basic rules of baseball

Kickball is a great way to introduce baseball rules to first graders. If you have eight or more, you can play regular kickball. Kickball rules are basically the same as baseball, except that the ball is pitched by rolling it across the plate (similar to bowling) and the ball is kicked rather than hit with a bat. It can be played inside or outside.

Variation: Mat Kickball is for eight or more players. You may have any number of people on a base. Base runner must round the bases twice before they can score. For example, before a runner can score he must go to first, second, third, first, second, third and then home. The only forced out is the kicker, if he does not reach first base before the ball. This keeps more people active during the game and avoids bored children on the bench. Gymnastic mats or rugs may be used as bases to allow more students to stand on the base. No leading off or stealing bases is allowed. Indoors the ball may be caught off the wall or ceiling for an out. A time limit of 5 minutes per side instead of three outs assures all students a chance to kick. The batting order will resume where it left off in the last inning. Indoors there are no out-of-bounds lines.

## 4. Fielding Drill

Equipment: 1 ball for each pair (tennis ball, softball)

Skill: fielding a ground ball

Pair students and have them roll a ball to each other and practice fielding a ground ball.

## 5. T-ball

Equipment: 1 bat, 1 ball, bases 20 to 30 feet apart depending upon age and facility

Skills: hitting, catching, fielding, throwing

Striking a pitched ball is very difficult. A good way to introduce striking for younger children is to have them hit a softball or waffle ball off a tee. Regular kickball or mat kickball rules may be used.

## 6. Waffle Ball

Equipment: 1 bat, 1 ball, bases
bases 20 to 30 feet apart depending upon age and facility

Skills: hitting, catching, fielding, throwing

Striking an underhand pitched ball is the next skill they should learn. Softball rules can be used. Mat kickball rules are recommended because it keeps more children active. At this level the teacher should do the pitching to assure the safety of the children. With older children (grades 4 and up), students may pitch, but they must pitch to their own teammates.

## 7. Work-up

Equipment: 1 bat, 1 ball, bases 20 to 30 feet apart depending upon age and facility

Skills: hitting, catching, fielding, throwing

Three students are batters. Seven to fourteen students are fielders. A batter stands at home plate and tries to get on base. If a fielder catches a fly ball, the fielder becomes a batter and the batter goes to right field. If a batter is tagged or forced out, then the batter goes to right field and all fielders rotate one position so the pitcher becomes a batter. Rotation is from right field, center field, left field, third base, second base, first base, pitcher, to batter. No score is kept. If all three batters are on base, then the one on third base is automatically out.

## Definition of Terms

**Base on Balls**—batter gains first base when the umpire judges four pitches to be balls.

**Base Line**—an imaginary line 3 feet to either side of a direct line between the bases.

**Batter's Box**—the area to which the batter is restricted while batting.

**Bunt**—a legal hit, intentionally tapped, ball that stays within the infield.

**Double Play**—a play by the defense in which two offensive players are legally put out.

**Force out**—an out in which the ball gets to a base before the base runner, and the base runner is forced to advance to the next base because the batter advances to first base.

**Infield Fly**—a fair, high fly ball that can be caught easily by an infielder and runners are on first, or first and second, or first, second, and third. The batter is automatically called out by the umpire even if the ball is dropped by the infielder. This rule is to protect base runners from the defense deliberately dropping a fly ball in order to gain a double play.

**Strike Zone**—the space over home plate which is between the batter's highest shoulder and his knees when the batter is in a natural batting stance.

**Legal Slow Pitch**—a pitch made from the hand below the hip that has a minimum arch of 3 feet and a maximum arch of 12 feet from the time it leaves the hand until it reaches the plate.

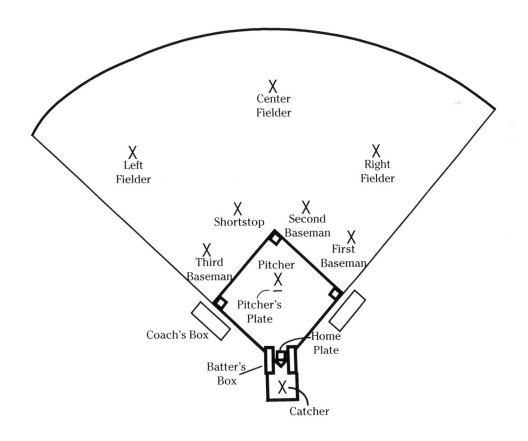

# LAB: OVERHAND THROW TECHNIQUE CHECKLIST
## (written for right hander)

Performer's Name _____ Age _____

Perform an overhand throw while someone observes you from the front, side, and back. The observer will look at one item from the checklist at a time and record a yes or no. Did you get "yes" for all the questions? If not, do it again, trying to correct your errors. (Younger children can use a smaller ball.) Videotape the person and have him use this checklist on himself.

## Overhand throw description:

The left side of the body faces in the direction you want to throw. Take a short step forward with the left foot. The elbow is the same height as the shoulder. Twist the shoulders and hips to the left as the arm swings forward. After the ball is released, step forward with the right foot. (A common error of young children is to have the wrong foot forward.)

## I. Stance

|  |  |  |  |
|---|---|---|---|
| **A.** | Are the feet shoulder width apart? | Yes | No |
| **B.** | Is a majority of the weight on the back foot? | Yes | No |
| **C.** | Is the left foot in front of the right foot in the direction of the throw? | Yes | No |
| **D.** | Is the left shoulder and hip pointing to the target? | Yes | No |
| **E.** | Is the non-throwing arm closest to the target? | Yes | No |
| **F.** | Is the trunk erect? | Yes | No |
| **G.** | Is the head up, erect, and eyes focused on the target? | Yes | No |

## II. Delivery
### TRUNK

|  |  |  |  |
|---|---|---|---|
| **A.** | Is the body straight at the waist? (trunk should not be bent at the waist) | Yes | No |
| **B.** | Are the shoulders level? | Yes | No |
| **C.** | At the beginning of the swing, are the shoulders and hips pointing in the direction the ball is intended to go? (A line drawn through both shoulders or hips should point to where the ball is intended to go.) | Yes | No |
| **D.** | At the conclusion of the swing, are the hips and shoulders facing the target? | Yes | No |

### FEET

|  |  |  |  |
|---|---|---|---|
| **E.** | Is a short step taken forward at the beginning of the throw? | Yes | No |
| **F.** | After the ball is released, does the right foot step forward? | Yes | No |

**Helpful phrase to say, "Focus your eyes on the target you are trying to hit."**

# LAB: BATTING
## TECHNIQUE CHECKLIST
### (written for right hander)

Performer's Name _____ Age _____

Bat a ball while someone observes you from the front, side, and back. The observer will look at one item from the checklist at a time and record a yes or no. Did you get "yes" for all the questions? If not, do it again, trying to correct your errors. (Younger children can use a rubber ball.) Videotape the person and have him use this checklist on himself.

## Batting description:

Select a bat that is appropriate to the age. Use an oversize plastic bat for ages 4 to 6. Use a short, light bat for ages 7 to 9. (Cut 4 to 5 inches off the end of a standard wood bat.) Stand with the left side toward the pitcher, with legs shoulder width apart. Grip the bottom of the handle with the left hand below the right hand and the hands touching. Both elbows should be 2 to 5 inches below the shoulder height and the bat held near the right shoulder. The bat should be vertical. After the ball is pitched, take a short step forward with the left foot. (If a child steps to the side instead of toward the pitcher, place a bench behind his legs. This will force him to step forward.) Rotate the hips and shoulders toward the pitcher. Swing the bat forward, keeping your eyes focused on the ball. The right heel will raise off the ground. After contacting the ball, continue to let the swing follow through and drop the bat (do not throw a bat.) The hips and shoulders should be facing the pitcher.

## I. Preparation

| | | | |
|---|---|---|---|
| **A.** | Is the left side toward the pitcher? | Yes | No |
| **B.** | Is the left hand on the bottom of the bat? | Yes | No |
| **C.** | Are the feet shoulder width apart? | Yes | No |
| **D.** | Are the shoulders level? | Yes | No |
| **E.** | Is the weight shifted to the back foot? | Yes | No |
| **F.** | Are the knees slightly flexed? | Yes | No |
| **G.** | Are the elbows approximately 2 to 5 inches below the height of the shoulders? | Yes | No |
| **H.** | Is the bat held to the rear as far as possible? | Yes | No |
| **I.** | Is the bat in a vertical position? | Yes | No |
| **J.** | Are the hands near the right shoulder? | Yes | No |
| **K.** | Are the wrists "snapped" forward as the bat meets the ball? | Yes | No |

## II. Action

| | | | |
|---|---|---|---|
| **A.** | Is a short step taken forward? | Yes | No |
| **B.** | Are the hips and shoulders rotating? | Yes | No |
| **C.** | Is the bat horizontal when it contacts the ball? | Yes | No |
| **D.** | Is the ball contacted in front of the front foot? | Yes | No |
| **E.** | Does the right heel raise off the ground? | Yes | No |
| **F.** | Are the eyes focused on the ball throughout the swing? | Yes | No |

## III. Follow-through

| | | | |
|---|---|---|---|
| **A.** | Does the bat continue to swing after contacting the ball? | Yes | No |
| **B.** | Do the hips face the pitcher? | Yes | No |

**Helpful phrase to say, "Watch the bat hit the ball."**

# VOLLEYBALL

Volleyball was invented by the YMCA in 1895 because a game was needed that a large number of men could play inside a gymnasium. The game used a tennis net strung high off the ground. It has become a popular recreational activity played by all ages.

## Basic Rules

The game is played by two teams of six players who attempt to hit the ball over the net and touch the opponent's floor inbounds for a score. When the ball is served, all players must be in their assigned positions. After the serve is contacted, the players may move anywhere on their side of the court.

### SERVING

The right back player is the server and must serve from behind the back base line and within the 10-foot serving area. The server serves until his side is out. The whole team rotates one position clockwise to determine the new server. A legal serve must go over the net without touching the net.

### VOLLEYING THE BALL

A player may hit the ball with any part of the body above the waist. After once contacting the ball, a player may not touch it again until it has been touched by some other player (exception is a block at the net. Any blocker may hit the ball a second time in a row.) A team has three hits to get the ball over the net.

### RESTRICTIONS OF BACKLINE PLAYERS

The back three players may not block a spike from the front 10 feet of the court.

### SCORING

One point is scored to the serving team if they win the serve. If the serving team loses the serve, no points are awarded. A game is played to 15 points and the winner must win by two points. A match is won by winning two out of three games.

### INFRACTIONS OF THE RULES

If a member of the receiving team commits an infraction, the serving team is awarded one point. If a member of the serving team commits an infraction, no points are awarded and the ball is given to the other team to serve. Infractions include:

(1) serving illegally; (2) touching the ball twice in a row; (3) touching the net; (4) a player's foot is completely in the opponent's court; (5) reaching under the net and touching an opponent; and (6) players being in the wrong positions during the serve.

## The Players

Players move to each position on the court throughout the course of a game. Teams are allowed up to six substitutions per match. However, substituted players may only return to the game in place of those teammates by whom they were replaced.

**The Server**—stands with both feet in the "service area" anywhere behind the baseline of the volleyball court. He or she tosses the ball in the air in front of his or her body, then strikes it with an open or closed hand or with the forearm. One player serves continuously until his or her team commits a "fault" resulting in a "side out," after which the opposite team "rotates" and serves the ball.

**Front-line Players (Left, Right, Middle)**—positioned in the frontcourt between the attack line and the net. These players mostly hit "spikes" into the opposite court and jump to "block" shots hit by the opposing side. Front-line players, while positioned in the frontcourt, may strike the ball when it is at any level above or below the net.

**Back-row Players (Left, Right, Middle Backs)**—play in the backcourt behind the attack line. They are primarily responsible for passing the ball toward teammates who then "set" the ball to other teammates in the attacking court for spikes. Back-row players also "dig" the ball on returned shots. While in the backcourt, these players may strike the ball when it is at any height above or below the net. However, if back-row players move over the attack line into the frontcourt, they may not strike the ball when it is above the height of the net. Therefore, they may not strike the ball as part of a blocking action.

## Basic Skills

Although volleyball requires few skills to learn, it is the most difficult game for children to learn. Volleyball is usually not taught until fourth or fifth grade because the children lack the coordination and strength to volley the ball accurately. By modifying the net height and serving distance, they can play the game.

There are two basic skills to volleyball. They are the serve and the passing or volley. Each of these two basic skills can be done overhand or underhand.

Stretch a rope across two chairs or trees if a regular net is not available.

1. **Wall Serve Drill**

   Equipment: 1 ball per student (Nerf, rubber ball, beach ball, or volleyball)

   Skills:  serving the volleyball

   Have the students stand approximately 8 feet from the wall and spaced 6 to 8 feet between students. The students will practice underhand serving into the wall. As they improve, have the students increase the distance from the wall.

   Variation—practice the overhand serve.

## Drills and Modified Games

| No. | Drill | Serve | Underhand Bump | Overhead Pass | Grade |
|-----|-------|-------|----------------|---------------|-------|
| 1. | Wall Serve Drill | x | | | 4–up |
| 2. | Wall Volley Drill | x | x | | 4–up |
| 3. | Circle Volley | | x | x | 4–up |
| 4. | Catch and Throw Volleyball | x | x | x | 4–up |

2. **Wall Volley Drill**

Equipment: 1 ball per student (Nerf, rubber ball, beach ball, or volleyball)

Skills: underhand bump and overhand pass

Have the students stand approximately 6 feet from the wall and spaced 6 to 8 feet between students. The students will practice hitting into the wall using the overhead pass and the underhand bump pass.

3. **Circle Volley**

Equipment: 1 ball per group (Nerf, rubber ball, beach ball, or volleyball)

Skills: underhand bump and overhead pass

Have three to four students form a circle 10 feet in diameter. The students will hit the ball to each other using the overhead pass and the underhand bump pass. Using beach balls will help the less skilled students learn the skill.

4. **Catch and Throw Volleyball**

Equipment: 1 ball

Skills: learn the rules

This game is good for beginners who are unskilled in hitting the ball. The ball may be caught and thrown over the net as well as hit over the net. A person may not take any steps while holding the ball. With mixed ages, the younger students are allowed to catch the ball and the older students must hit the ball.

Variation—Play with two or three balls.

5. **Beach ball Volleyball**

Equipment: 1 or 2 beach balls

Skills: all skills

A volleyball game is played with a beach ball. The server will have to stand close to the net in order to get the ball over. The beach ball travels slower and allows less skilled players to participate.

Variation—Play with two beach balls. Each team serves one ball at the same time. The first ball to touch the floor loses the point. This allows twice as many students to participate. It is helpful if more than six players are on a team.

# LAB: VOLLEYBALL OVERHEAD PASS TECHNIQUE CHECKLIST

Performer's Name _____ Age _____

    Perform an overhead pass while someone observes you from the front, side, and back. The observer will look at one item from the checklist at a time and record a yes or no. Did you get "yes" for all the questions? If not, do it again, trying to correct your errors. (Younger children can use a smaller ball.) Videotape the person and have him use this checklist on himself.

## Overhead pass description:

    The overhead pass is the primary pass used to handle balls that are above the chest. The overhead pass is accurate and is often used for setting the ball for a spike. Bend the knees slightly with the feet in a front-to-back positioning. The elbows are out to the side, at approximately shoulder height. The fingers and thumbs should be 2 to 3 inches apart and 2 to 3 inches from the forehead. The player should watch the ball through the "window" created by the fingers and thumbs. When the ball is 2 to 3 inches from the hands, fully extend the elbows and hit the ball with stiff fingers. Catching the ball is not allowed. Often children are not coordinated enough to do this skill until grade 4.

## I. Preparation
### LEGS

|   |   |   |   |
|---|---|---|---|
| **A.** | Is the body facing the direction the ball is coming from? | Yes | No |
| **B.** | Is one foot ahead of the other? | Yes | No |
| **C.** | Are the knees slightly flexed? | Yes | No |

### ELBOWS

|   |   |   |   |
|---|---|---|---|
| **D.** | Are the elbows pointed out to the sides? | Yes | No |
| **E.** | Are the elbows approximately shoulder height? | Yes | No |

### HANDS

|   |   |   |   |
|---|---|---|---|
| **F.** | Are the hands 2 to 3 inches above the forehead? | Yes | No |
| **G.** | Are the fingers and thumbs 2 to 3 inches apart? | Yes | No |

## II. Action

|   |   |   |   |
|---|---|---|---|
| **A.** | Are the eyes focused on the ball at all times? | Yes | No |
| **B.** | Is the ball hit with the thumbs and fingers? | Yes | No |
| **C.** | Are the fingers "stiff" during the hit? | Yes | No |
| **D.** | Is there full extension of the elbow, shoulder, and body? | Yes | No |

**Helpful phrase to say, "Watch the ball through the window you made."**

# LAB: VOLLEYBALL BUMP
# TECHNIQUE CHECKLIST
## (written for right hander)

Performer's Name _____ Age _____

    Perform an underhand bump while someone observes you from the front, side, and back. The observer will look at one item from the checklist at a time and record a yes or no. Did you get "yes" for all the questions? If not, do it again, trying to correct your errors. (Younger children can use a smaller ball.) Videotape the person and have him use this checklist on himself.

## Volleyball bump description:

    The two-hand underhand hit (bump) is used when the ball is below the waist. The ball is bounced off the forearms. Place the right hand on top of the left hand with palms up. Place the right thumb on top of the left thumb. Stand with the feet in a front-to-back position. Have the knees flexed and the hands below the waist. As the ball approaches, keep the elbow as close as possible to each other. Let the ball rebound off the forearms. Often children do not have the coordination to do the bump until grade 4.

## I. Preparation

    **A.** Is one foot ahead of the other?     Yes     No
    **B.** Are the feet in a front-to-back position?     Yes     No
    **C.** Is the right hand on top of the left and palms up?     Yes     No
    **D.** Is the right thumb on top of the left thumb?     Yes     No
    **E.** Are the elbows almost touching each other?     Yes     No
    **F.** Are the knees bent?     Yes     No
    **G.** Are the hands below the waist?     Yes     No

## II. Action

    **A.** Are the eyes watching the ball at all times?     Yes     No
    **B.** Is the ball hit by the lower, inner forearm?     Yes     No
    **C.** Do the arms move slightly up to hit the ball?     Yes     No

**Helpful phrase to say, "Watch the ball hit your forearms."**

# LAB: UNDERHAND SERVE
## TECHNIQUE CHECKLIST
### (written for right hander)

Performer's Name _____ Age _____

Perform an underhand serve, while someone observes you from the front, side, and back. The observer will look at one item from the checklist at a time and record a yes or no. Did you get "yes" for all the questions? If not, do it again, trying to correct your errors. (Younger children can use a smaller ball.) Videotape the person and have him use this checklist on himself.

## Serve description:

The underhand serve is the easiest to learn but is not as powerful as the overhand serve. Stand facing the net with the left foot forward and bend the body slightly forward from the waist. Hold the ball in the left hand at waist height in front of the left foot. Hold the right arm in a back position behind the right hip. Swing the right arm forward and shift the weight from the right foot to the left foot. The hand should be palm toward the ball and the ball is struck at the base of the hand or "heel of the hand." The eyes should be focused on the middle of the ball at all times. Start by hitting the ball off the hand, then progress to tossing the ball slightly before you strike it.

## I. Preparation

| | | | |
|---|---|---|---|
| **A.** | Is one foot ahead of the other? | Yes | No |
| **B.** | Are the knees slightly bent? | Yes | No |
| **C.** | Is the body slightly bent forward at the waist? | Yes | No |
| **D.** | Is the ball held at waist height? | Yes | No |

## II. Action

| | | | |
|---|---|---|---|
| **A.** | Is the ball struck with the heel of the hand? | Yes | No |
| **B.** | Are the eyes focused on the ball? | Yes | No |
| **C.** | Is the weight shifted from the back foot to the front foot? | Yes | No |
| **D.** | Does the arm follow-through straight ahead? | Yes | No |
| | (The arm should not go sideways.) | | |

**Helpful phrase to say, "Watch the hand strike the middle of the ball."**

# TENNIS

## History

A game similar to tennis was played by French kings and noblemen in the sixteenth and seventeenth centuries. Folklore says two English visitors to France watched the game and heard the word *tenez* which means, "resume play." They took the name and game of tennis back to England. Lawn tennis was patented in 1873 by Major Wingfield in England. Today tennis is played by all ages and is a good aerobic activity.

## Terminology

**Ace**—a serve where the tennis ball served is served in and not touched by the receiver.

**Ad In**—the score when the player serving wins the point when the score is at deuce.

**Ad Out**—the score when the receiving player wins the point when the score is at deuce.

**Advantage**—when one player wins a point from a deuce and needs one more point to win the game.

**All**—the score is tied (example: 30 all means the score is tied at 30–30.)

**Backcourt**—the area on the court between the rear baseline and the service line.

**Baseline**—the chalk line at the farthest ends of the court indicating the boundary of the area of play.

**Cross Court**—hitting the ball diagonally from one side of the court to the other.

**Deuce**—tie score of 40–40. A player must win two consecutive points from a deuce before winning the game.

**Double Fault**—two successive faults by the server, causing the server to lose the point.

**Doubles**—a game where four people play two on each side as partners.

**Fault**—a serve that fails to place the ball in the correct area of play.

**Let**—a served ball touches the net and goes into the proper court; it is played again.

**Lob**—a ball is hit with a high arc, sometimes done to hit over an opponent who is at the net.

**Love**—a scoring term meaning no point.

**Out**—a ball that touches the ground outside of the boundary lines. A ball that touches the line is considered in play.

**Serve**—the opening hit of each point begins with the server standing beyond the back line and hitting the ball into the appropriate court.

**Volley**—hitting the ball before it touches the ground.

## Scoring

Scoring in tennis is unusual. The server's score is called first.

| | |
|---|---|
| 0 points | love |
| 1st point | 15 |
| 2nd point | 30 |
| 3rd point | 40 |
| 4th point | game |

Deuce means that each side has scored three points or more and is tied. You must win by two points. The first point after deuce is called advantage. If the server has the point, it is called ad in. If the receiver has the advantage, it is called ad out.

## A PLAYER LOSES THE POINT WHEN:

- The player does a double fault.
- The player does not return the ball into the playing court.
- The player touches the ball more than once with his racquet while making a stroke. In doubles only one of the players may hit the ball.
- The player hits the ball before it has passed over the net.
- The ball hits the player or his clothing.
- The player throws his racquet at the ball.

## Gripping the racquet

When doing a forehand stroke the "V" formed by the thumb and index finger will be on top of the racquet with the face of the racquet perpendicular to the ground.

When doing a backhand stroke, rotate the racquet one quarter turn to the left. This will keep the racquet face perpendicular to the ground while hitting the ball.

## Strategy

Standing at the rear baseline in the middle is best. If your opponent hits a short shot, then you can rush to the net to hit the return shot. Standing in the center of the court is the worst place to be. The ball will land at your feet and be difficult to hit.

# LAB: TENNIS FOREHAND
## TECHNIQUE CHECKLIST
### (written for right hander)

Performer's Name _____ Age _____

    Perform a forehand stroke while someone observes you from the front, side, and back. The observer will look at one item from the checklist at a time and record a yes or no. Did you get "yes" for all the questions? If not, do it again, trying to correct your errors. (Younger children can use a racquetball racquet.) Videotape the person and have him use this checklist on himself.

## Forehand swing description:

    Grip the racquet handle in the manner of a handshake. The palm should be on the back side of the racquet handle. The "V" notch formed by the thumb and index finger should be pointed toward the edge of the racquet. The thumb should not be on the top of the handle. The racquet should be pointed toward the back fence at waist height and arm straight. The trunk of the body should be facing the side fence. To initiate the swing, step toward the ball with the front foot. Keep your weight on the balls of the feet. Simultaneously rotate the hips and swing the arm, keeping it straight. The ball should be contacted in a plane with the front foot and the head of the racquet held vertical. Watch the ball at all times as you swing. In the follow-through, the wrist is kept firm at all times. The racquet will be brought past the left eye. In order to keep the arm straight while swinging, you must position your body so that the ball is farther than arms-length from you.

## I. Grip

    **A.** Is the V notch of the thumb and index finger on the edge
of the racket?                         Yes     No

## II. Feet

    **A.** Is the front (left) heel rising off the court during the swing?   Yes     No
    **B.** Is the front foot stepping toward the net?
    **C.** Is the front foot twisting on the ball of the foot during
the swing?                               Yes     No
    **D.** Is the right foot coming up on the toe and sole of the foot
facing the rear fence after the shot?            Yes     No

## III. Trunk

    **A.** Are the shoulders level?                      Yes     No

**B.** Are the hips twisting during the shot and ending up
   facing the net?                                      Yes      No
**C.** Is the body upright at the waist?                Yes      No
   (Trunk should not be bent at the waist.)

## IV. Swing

**A.** Does the racquet swing follow through and point in the
   direction the ball is intended to go?               Yes      No
**B.** Is only one hand holding the racquet?            Yes      No
**C.** Do the eyes see the ball contact the racquet?    Yes      No

## V. Racket Position

**A.** Is the wrist at eye level at the end of the swing?       Yes      No
**B.** Is the tip of the racquet pointing in the direction of the hit?   Yes      No
**C.** Is the elbow in front of the chin at the end of the swing?   Yes      No
**D.** Is the racket turned over with the face pointing to the
   ground?                                              Yes      No
**E.** Is the elbow relatively straight throughout the swing?   Yes      No

**Helpful phrase to say, "Watch the ball hit the strings."**

# LAB: TENNIS BACKHAND
# TECHNIQUE CHECKLIST
(written for right hander)

Performer's Name _____ Age _____

Perform a backhand stroke while someone observes you from the front, side, and back. The observer will look at one item from the checklist at a time and record a yes or no. Did you get "yes" for all the questions? If not, do it again, trying to correct your errors. (Younger children can use a racquetball racquet.) Videotape the person and have him use this checklist on himself.

## Backhand swing description:

Grip the racquet with a forehand grip. Rotate the hand one quarter turn until the palm is on top edge of the racquet handle. The "V" notch will be on the front side of the racquet. Turn the body until it faces sideways to the net. The knees are bent and the eyes are looking at the ball over the right shoulder. A short step is taken forward with the right foot as the swing is initiated. The ball is contacted slightly ahead of the front foot, the elbow fully extended. The racquet face is vertical when it contacts the ball. The eyes should focus on the ball at all times. The backhand may be done with one or two hands. Younger children should use two hands when they lack the strength to get the ball to the net. Children ages 6 to 8 do not have the strength to swing a tennis racquet and should be given a racquetball racquet to learn with.

## I. Grip

**A.** Is the knuckle of the index finger on the top edge of the racquet? (If the ball goes high into the air, then the grip is possibly wrong.)                                    Yes          No

## II. Feet

**A.** Is the front foot stepping toward the net?                    Yes          No
**B.** Is the front foot pointing in the direction the ball is to go?   Yes          No
**C.** Is the back foot coming to the very tip of the toe at the conclusion of the swing?                                  Yes          No
**D.** Are the ball and racket meeting at a point in front of the body and not behind the body?                          Yes          No

## III. Trunk

| | | | |
|---|---|---|---|
| **A.** | Is the body straight at the waist? (trunk should not be bent at the waist) | Yes | No |
| **B.** | Are the shoulders level? | Yes | No |
| **C.** | At the beginning of the swing, are the shoulders and hips pointing in the direction the ball is intended to go? (A line drawn through both shoulders or hips should point to where the ball is intended to go.) | Yes | No |
| **D.** | At the conclusion of the swing, are the hips and shoulders facing the direction the ball is to go? | Yes | No |

## IV. Swing

| | | | |
|---|---|---|---|
| **A.** | Is the tip of the racquet pointing in the direction of the hit? | Yes | No |
| **B.** | Is only one hand holding the racquet? | Yes | No |
| **C.** | Do the eyes see the ball contacting the racquet? | Yes | No |

## V. Racquet Position

| | | | |
|---|---|---|---|
| **A.** | Is the elbow relatively straight throughout the swing? | Yes | No |
| **B.** | Is the wrist eye level ? | Yes | No |
| **C.** | Are the ball and racquet meeting at a point in front of the body and not behind the body? | Yes | No |

**Helpful phrase to say, "Watch the ball hit the strings."**

## ULTIMATE FRISBEE

### History

While the exact origins of Ultimate Frisbee are uncertain, it is believed that high school teenagers in Maplewood, New Jersey, were the first to invent and play the game, initially as an evening pastime in 1968. The rules we have today are the same as in 1968. The game quickly spread worldwide as a fun aerobic recreational game for all ages. Teams can compete in national and international competition.

Ultimate Frisbee is a non-contact team sport that is a combination of football and soccer but using a Frisbee instead of a ball. It combines the nonstop movement and athletic endurance of soccer with the passing skills of football. Ultimate Frisbee is played on a football field with seven players on each team. The object of the game is to score by catching a pass in the opponent's end zone, similar to football or rugby. Players may not run while holding the Frisbee, but may pivot and pass to any of the other receivers on the field. Receivers run pass patterns similar to football, but play never stops, like soccer. After a point is scored, play resumes from the end zone where the point was scored. Ultimate tournaments have no referees. The players are responsible to govern the game play in a spirit of good sportsmanship. In recreational games, the number of players may vary and the field is smaller.

### Change of Possession

An incomplete pass results in a change of possession. When this happens the defense immediately becomes the offense and gains possession of the Frisbee where it comes to a stop on the playing field or where it traveled out-of-bounds.

Reasons for turnovers:

- **Throw-away**—The thrower misses his target and the disc falls to the ground.
- **Drops**—The receiver is not able to catch the disc.
- **Blocks**—A defender deflects the disc in midflight, causing it to hit the ground.
- **Interceptions**—A defender catches a disc thrown by the offense.
- **Out-of-bounds**—The disc lands out-of-bounds, hits an object out-of-bounds, or is caught by a player who lands or leaps from outside the playing field.
- **Stalls**—A player on offense does not release the disc after the defender has counted out 10 seconds.

### Fouls

A foul is the result of contact between players, although incidental contact (not affecting the play) does not constitute a foul. When a foul disrupts possession, possession of the Frisbee is given to the offended team. Stripping the Frisbee away from a player is considered a foul.

### Offensive Strategies

A common offensive strategy is the **vertical stack**. In this strategy, the offense lines up in a straight line along the length of the field. From this position, players in the stack make sudden sprints out of the stack towards or away from the thrower in an attempt to get open and receive the disc.

Another offensive strategy is the **horizontal stack.** Three throwers line up across the width of the field with four receivers upfield, also lined up across the field. If no upfield options are available, the thrower swings the disc side to side in an attempt to reset the stall count while also getting the defense out of position.

## Defensive Strategies

One strategy is for each defender to cover one receiver (one on one.) Another strategy is zone. In a zone defense each player covers a predetermined area of the playing field instead of a player. The player defending the thrower should aggressively attempt to block the throw.

## Throwing the Frisbee

There are two major grips used to throw a disc—backhand and forehand.

**Backhand:** Grip the Frisbee so that all your fingers are wrapped around the edge of the frisbee and your thumb lies along the top of the disc. With the disc level, extend the throwing arm across your body and swing your arm away from your body, releasing the disc when your arm is about 45 degrees from your body with a snap of the wrist. At the same time, step forward with your right leg;

you should complete your step and release the disc at approximately the same time. The power behind your throw should come mostly from wrist motion and partly from the movement of your arm.

**Forehand:** The forehand throw is more difficult and takes practice. Grip the disc with two fingers and the thumb. Place your middle finger on the rim of the underside of the disc. Extend your index finger toward the center of the disc on the underside and rest your thumb on the top of the disc, wrapping it around the edge. The power behind the forehand throw comes almost completely from your wrist. Stand with the disc to your right (right handers,) horizontal to the ground. Hold it slightly behind your body. Rotate the disc on your wrist behind your hand and snap your wrist forward, moving your arm forward slightly also. Release the disc when your arm and wrist movement brings it in front of you about 45 degrees. At the same time, step forward with your right foot, stepping down just as you release the disc.

# APPENDIX

# Height & Weight Chart

School Year _____

| Names | | | | | |
|-------|---|---|---|---|---|
| September | | | | | |
| October | | | | | |
| November | | | | | |
| December | | | | | |
| January | | | | | |
| February | | | | | |
| March | | | | | |
| April | | | | | |
| May | | | | | |
| June | | | | | |
| July | | | | | |
| August | | | | | |

# Suggested Equipment Needs

Below is a list of suggested equipment for the lesson plans and home use. Keep in mind that buying used equipment can greatly reduce costs.

Bean bags

Mini Nerf basketball, 4" diameter

Nerf basketball, 6"–8" diameter (Grades K–3)

Junior Sizes basketball (Grades 3–4

Girl's Size basketball (Grades 4–6)

Boy's Size basketball (Grades 6–up)

Rubber utility ball, 8" diameter

Wiffle ball, bat, tee

Baseball glove (Grades 2–up)

Tennis balls

Racquetball racquet

Tennis racquet (Grades 4–up)

Jump ropes

25 feet Sash cord or clothes line 3/8" or 1/2"

Board 2x4 or 4x4 ten feet long (balance beam)

Hula Hoop

Exercise mat

Hoppity Hop 14" diameter (ages 2–6)

Inner tube

Rope, 1" diameter 12' long (climbing rope)

Iron pipe 1.5"–2", diameter 10' long (fireman pole)

Rubber ball 34

Rubber ball 21

Mini trampoline

Milk cartons, Plastic five gallon pail, Plastic trash can

# Quick Reference Guide for Exercise-Related Injuries

| Injury | Symptoms | Prevention | Treatment |
|---|---|---|---|
| **Blisters** | Raised area where fluid collects under skin | Wear two pairs of socks | Avoid puncturing. If painful, clean area and carefully drain blister. Protect area with sterile dressing |
| **Heat Exhaustion** | Skin is pale, cool and moist due to recent exposure to high temperatures | Drink water before exercise, and take water breaks while exercising. Do not take salt tablets | Get to a cool area and cool the body as much as possible |
| **Heatstroke** | Skin is hot and dry and body does not sweat. Dizziness or weakness | Drink water before exercise, and take water breaks while exercising | This is a medical emergency. Cool the body as fast as possible and get victim to the hospital |
| **Joint Sprain** | Pain, tenderness, and swelling near the joint | Warm up before exercise. Work to strengthen muscles over the long term | Rest. Elevate the injury, wrap in an elastic bandage, and apply ice |
| **Muscle Cramp** | Sharp pains in the muscles (usually the legs) | Rest. Prevent by taking calcium supplements | Gently stretch the muscle |
| **Shin splints** | Pain in the front part of the lower leg | Warm-up before exercise and increase length and intensity of work out gradually instead of suddenly. Work to strengthen muscles over the long term. Wear good shoes with a firm heel. Avoid running on hard surfaces | Rest and ice the area |
| **Tendonitis/Tennis Elbow** | Pain in the joint | Warm-up before exercise. Work to strengthen muscles over the long term. Avoid overuse | Rest. Elevate the injury and wrap in an elastic bandage. Take ibuprofen to reduce swelling |

# Aerobic Ball Exercises

## Rainy days and cold winter days

Have you wondered what to do with your energetic children when they can't go outside? These simple exercises are a great solution! Plus, they provide a superior balance and exercise workout because they utilize almost all of the muscles of the body, all at the same time. That means you get the effect of a high impact aerobic routine with very little actual impact. Plus, it's fun! (Trust me: children love this one!)

These routines require a 21" rubber or vinyl inflatable ball (26" ball for older children or adults and 18" or 21" ball for younger children). These exercises are appropriate for any age, as long as the child can sit on a ball without falling off (usually, that means ages 6 and up; younger children tend to get a little wild and bounce off the ball too much).

Be sure and choose a safe area, clear of sharp corners or big objects, to avoid injury when your child bounces off the ball.

This routine takes about 15 minutes to complete.

## The Routine

Begin by sitting on the ball. The knees should be bent at a 90 degree angle (the ball can be inflated or deflated slightly to accomplish this.) Be sure to progress in the order provided below, so that the skill level is appropriate.

**Warm-up**—Begin by gently bouncing on the ball. As you get the feel of the rhythm, let your arms swing alternately forward and back (gently to start). Gradually increase the swing until you are bouncing fairly vigorously. Bounce for at least 3 minutes as a warm-up.

**Alternate Arms And Legs**—While bouncing, kick out the right leg with the left arm, then the left leg with the right arm (similar to a vigorous walking motion.)

**Hopping In Circles**—With arms out to the side for balance, sit on the ball and hop around in a circle.

**Side Kicks**—With arms out to the side for balance, bounce. Then bring both feet to alternate sides of the ball, while continuing to bounce.

**Sit Ups**—Position the hips a little further back on the ball (you will need to "feel" the position that is right). Lean forward and touch your toes, then sit back up and reach backwards with arms over the head until you are touching the floor behind your head. Repeat. (The trick is to get balanced on the ball in the correct spot. It's not as hard as it sounds!)

**Flying**—Keeping hips on the ball, roll onto your stomach. Keep the toes on the floor and raise the arms overhead 10 to 20 times (no bouncing needed).

**Foot Rolls**—Still on your stomach, roll forward on the ball until just the lower legs and feet are on the ball (about one foot apart). Keep your hands on the floor. Roll the ball side to side with your feet.

**Roll The Ball**–Climb on top of the ball, on your hands and kneels. Roll the ball the length of the room without touching the ground.

**Return To The Warm-up**—for at least 3 minutes when done. This is the "cool down" process.

# ABOUT THE AUTHOR

DR. BRUCE WHITNEY received his Ph.D. from the University of Minnesota School of Kinesiology. He and his wife Lynn have nine children, and they have home educated their children since 1987.

Dr. Whitney's professional experiences include teaching at the elementary, secondary, and college levels. His responsibilities have included being an intramural director, a day camp director, and a coach for a variety of sports for students ranging from elementary through collegiate levels. As a college professor he was involved in training future teachers in physical education. He also gained a cross-cultural perspective on sport and fitness while teaching at the University of the Philippines, Manila. He has taught physical education in three home school co-ops. He has been a guest speaker at state home-school conventions. His insights come from years of teaching experience as a professional and as a parent.

Dr. Whitney is presently an adjunct professor at Anoka Ramsey Community College in Coon Rapids, Minnesota.

## Editorial Assistant and Exercise Consultant

Sherrie Lange has worked as a physical therapist since 1977 and is also a home school mom.

# Resources

## WEBSITES

**American Alliance for Health, Physical Education and Dance (AAHPERD)**
www.aahperd.org
An alliance of five national associations and six district associations that provides a variety of resources.

**Amateur Athletic Union**
www.aausports.org
Sponsors a variety of youth sports.

**California Education Department**
www.cde.ca.gov/ci/pe/cf/
Physical Education Model Content Standards for California Public Schools

**Can Do Videotapes**
www.candokids.com
Exercise videos by home school children which include memorizing math facts while you exercise.

**Canadian Association for Health, Physical Education, Recreation and Dance (CAHPERD)**
www.cahperd.ca
Recommended Physical Education Standards

**Cooper Institute**
www.cooperinst.org
Dr. Cooper's web site with research information

**Fitnessgram Tests**
www.fitnessgram.net

**Home School Family Fitness Institute**
hsffi.com
physical education books and videos

**Kanakuk-Kanakomo Kamps**
www.kanakuk.com
Christian Athletic Camps

**The National Association for Sport and Physical Education (NASPE)**
National Standards for Physical Education

**PE Central**
www.pecentral.org
lesson plans and equipment

**President's Challenge**
President's Council on Physical Fitness and Sports
www.presidentschallenge.org
www.fitness.gov
Students who score in the top 15% of all the fitness tests will receive the Presidential Physical Fitness Award

**YMCA of the USA**
www.ymca.net
Develops national programs and publishes books in youth fitness and sports. Provides facilities and programs for infants to seniors in branches all across the USA. Programs include youth sports.

## BOOKS, ARTICLES AND JOURNALS

*A Manual For Tumbling and Apparatus Stunts* by Ryser and Brown, Wm. C. Brown Publishers, 1990
Excellent instructional manual for gymnastics

*The Journal of the American Medical Association*
http://jama.ama-assn.org/

*Generation M: Media in the Lives of 8–18 Year Olds* by Dr. Donald F. Roberts, Ulla G. Foehr, and Victoria Rideout
The Kaiser Family Foundation, 2005
www.kff.org

*Kid Fitness* by Kenneth H. Cooper, Bantam Books, 1992

*The Ultimate Homeschool Physical Education Game Book* by Guy Baily, Educators Press, 2003
www.educatorspress.com
A book of games modified to be played with a limited number of children

*Moving Into the Future: National Physical Education Standards*
National Association for Sport and Physical Education
www.aapherd.org/naspe

*Research Quarterly for Exercise and Sport*
A professional journal offering the latest research in the art and science of human movement studies.

*YMCA Physical Fitness Handbook* by Clayton R. Myers; Nick Cardy, Warner Books, 1975

## OTHER

**U.S. Department of Education**
For the research study called "First Lessons: A Report on Elementary Education in America"